WILD
HEART

HEALTHY LIFE

When the Odds are Against You,
Your Lifestyle Matters

Melissa Viator

AuthorHouse™
1663 Liberty Drive
Bloomington, IN 47403
www.authorhouse.com
Phone: 1 (800) 839-8640

Published by AuthorHouse 05/07/2019

ISBN: 978-1-5462-7804-7 (sc)
ISBN: 978-1-5462-7805-4 (e)

Library of Congress Control Number: 2019901056

Print information available on the last page.

This book is printed on acid-free paper.

authorHOUSE®

DEDICATION

To my beloved children, to help them become compassionate for other people and their environment, make better food choices, and learn to always find positivity in their lives. I hope to inspire a healthier lifestyle for them and anyone who reads this despite their obstacles in life.

To my family, who has given me much to think about throughout my life. You have set the foundation for my thoughts and forced me to process emotions and accept and love family members for who they are.

To my husband, who always supports my most challenging ambitions and continues to love me unconditionally through it all.

CONTENTS

PROLOGUE

This book will resonate with everyone in some way or another. The topics are close to home and will make you think about your own personal habits, behaviors, and people in your life. I needed to write this book to open up a sensitive dialogue on topics we just cannot clearly describe in their entirety and that are often left unspoken as undefined mysteries about ourselves that hold much meaning. Here, we will conceptualize personal questions like why we have interchangeable moods, highs and lows, and feelings of worthlessness at times. These feelings can waste our precious time, and I want us to enjoy life to its fullest.

I use my own life experiences to set the stage for your personal explorations, all while avoiding comparison and judgment. Comparing your life with others' and judging them is a waste of time and evidence of a weak backbone – so to speak. And so, I leave judgment at the door but open my wild heart for you to resonate with and to learn that you are never alone in this world. Judgment is a form of clear evidence that you are insecure about your own fears and uncertainties. Likewise, it creates obstacles that delay a healthy lifestyle. It stops you from being the best—well, *person* you absolutely can be. I'm providing my examples as a tool for you to use in doing your own deep thinking as you closely evaluate your lifestyle for what it truly means and how it affects you. This is a book that will influence you to delve deeply into your own food habits and social environment and learn where it all stems from on a personal level. It will make you cry and hopefully laugh. It will help you make better life choices that support feeling the very best you can possible be. It will help you become more balanced mentally, socially, and emotionally. It will help you learn to be more human and develop the courage to love yourself for who you are.

I'll start by letting you in on my very own important secret that literally shaped me into who I am today. I'm guilty of living with the Viking mentality—that is, kill or be killed. I am great at building a bulletproof shell around myself and living a numb existence to ensure I will never be vulnerable. I refuse to be victimized and always wear a mask that conveys, "No one will ever be welcome inside my head or learn my weaknesses." In time, I realized this Viking mentality was a means of survival by creating a false dichotomy in which, if I don't do the crushing, I will fall prey to my own environment.

This is how I remember how I got through my childhood. My mentality ran parallel with the Vikings' on the battlefield. It defined the untouchable, unbreakable, and confident character I wanted to portray. I wore thick armor and felt invincible. In truth, I was in survival mode as a child. Although this way of surviving was not a healthy way to continue to live, it had indeed shaped my adult habits and behaviors that suppressed my way of living altogether. I'll explain more details in a bit as it took some time to learn how to release the Viking inside me. It took time to realize that I need love, growth, and renewal to truly live a healthy and balanced life. It literally took decades to figure this out, and here I am now writing to you to explain that strength does not come from the experiences we live through; it comes with the human connection we feel with others during those experiences. I am here to explain that you need vulnerability, courage, and kindness to grow within, and it all stems from our wild hearts. Our hearts are like wild animals thriving instinctively. We all know right from wrong in some capacity, but our environments influence us to make decisions, ultimately, on how we conduct ourselves in social interactions, make food choices, and handle outcomes that originated from our past experiences.

Decisions are perhaps the only aspect of your life that you are truly in control of. In my experiences, I have found that criticism is a form of self-protection, in terms of protecting myself from feeling fear and worthlessness. It was so easy for me to criticize and judge others because, in reality, I feared knowing and accepting the truth about my own faults and imperfections. I feared not being good enough my whole life, as I am sure you may have had similar insecurities from one time or another. Instead of feeling sorry for myself and binge eating or drinking, I thought about how I could make contributions in society or, at the very least, appreciate others' achievements. It is a risk to throw your authentic self out there just to be scrutinized and judged. But nothing positive ever comes from criticizing one's actions or passing judgment. Even if a nasty, yet clever, defensive response feels amazing for a split second, it is quickly forgotten and leaves you feeling empty—shameful, even. Shame makes you feel completely irrelevant and unable to handle rapid change and contribute to society. It will literally cause delays in your personal growth and open doors for a destructive lifestyle or, at best, poor eating habits. This book will open other doors for people living within their darkest days. Subtle life changes can make a huge difference in your quality of life, and so I needed to publish a manuscript that provides an example for others to help make these subtle changes. Food choices and food preparation methods can make a huge difference in your mood, social environment, and long-term health.

I wanted to write a book that shares a heartfelt childhood that led me to the path to a particular lifestyle. This book shares my story of the adverse childhood and military experiences I had all while beating the odds for the very best and healthiest outcome. It explains how we can break the cycles of substance abuse, domestic abuse, chronic disease, and low socioeconomic status if we know how to identify and understand certain factors in our lives, and it bridges the gap between how we were raised and the adults we are capable of becoming through food choices and our social environment.

I would not be completely honest with you by saying that only negative outcomes came from my childhood. That is not what this book is about and it could not be more opposite from the truth. Some of my best qualities are based on *all* of my childhood experiences and, for the most part, came from my parents, siblings, and close friends, including the way I love people; the way I care for people who are having their absolute worst days; the way I can empathize for those hurting and laugh until I pee myself in the same breath, which happens pretty often; the way I have learned to truly understand people before my opinions even have a chance to develop; the way I stop and think about a homeless person or someone with different abilities and know they have an interesting story to tell; the way I can understand that all people have different body types and food behaviors that originally manifested from their environments or perhaps their cultures.

Instead of asking questions like, "Why am I living like this?" or "What the hell is wrong with me?" ask the question, "What happened?" instead. Understanding the core roots of your personal development will answer the mysteries of yourself and the life choices you have made.

Food choices, environments, and socioeconomic conversations are tangible in the sense that we can actually feel the difference that food choices have on us, we can visibly see our environments and make the decision to leave or change them, and we can mentally and physically set goals to reach a higher socioeconomic status. We can tangibly make an honest effort to become better versions of ourselves. We cannot, on the other hand, fully explain why we have certain moods and feelings of uncertainty. Even if we have learned the tools to complete self-love, there will always be moments of uncertainty that just throw our day, or perhaps week, completely off.

If you only remember one message from reading this book, I hope it has something to do with learning how to love and accept yourself completely. I hope you learn to be more mindful of everything you are absolutely capable of becoming without letting imperfections and insecurities hold you back. I hope you learn to find the courage to absolutely love your life and know you have the simple tools to make it healthier.

Nothing is discredited in this book. Nothing is judged, and opinionated statements are a waste of your time, as well as mine. Learning to accept the person I have become has been the hardest concept to swallow, but it is the most important message to convey. You would think that if I was so passionate about this topic that it should be the easiest thing to talk about, right? Well, not necessarily. It took courage to expose my own wild heart, so be kind.

ACKNOWLEDGMENTS

How could I write this book without acknowledging the people who gave me the courage to speak up and drive on every single day? The countless hours of deep conversations and unstoppable tears were the best therapy throughout my childhood and are still my heartbeat in my life today. I owe my closest friends, my sister, and my husband the utmost gratitude for listening to me when I was in my darkest moments. I am so grateful for the people in my life who constantly gave their unconditional love and became my personal psychotherapists in many ways than one—those who would never pass judgment and always provided a safe space for me to be absolutely honest when I needed to talk through my feelings and concerns. Those who witnessed my most vulnerable moments and my most depressed state of mind, knowing that my phone call would probably suck up at least an hour of their time. Still, they continued to show up just to listen to me. I am most grateful for them always providing me with the "voice of reason," which they all continue to lend me. And for that, I want to publicly acknowledge them in this book as a reminder to everyone that we cannot do anything alone. Strength does not come from the experiences we live through; it comes with the human connection we feel with others during those experiences. I am forever grateful for the people in my life, family and friends alike, who have shaped my view of the morals, values, and beliefs I hold dearly.

INTRODUCTION

Can you imagine a life that is full of choices that optimize your ability to live a healthy lifestyle? Did you ever wonder why you suddenly feel depressed but don't know any reason to feel that way? Are you raising little ones in your home who absolutely need the same nutritional, balanced diet as you? After a decade of conceptualizing my own personal misunderstood moods, I began to delve deeper into what lifestyle I have evolved into. I studied all things I consumed (e.g., food, alcohol, drugs) and the environment to which I was exposed in my life from infancy until today. Our lives are full of choices that alter our moods, which are essentially rooted in the food we eat and the social experiences in which we take part. Adverse childhood experiences, or ACEs, are becoming a common subject of study that explains the connection of specific unexplainable mood triggers that are linked to significant childhood events. Hence, it should be no surprise that our lifelong environments and exposures write our personal stories. Simultaneously, our diets affect our moods and, eventually, our long-term health as well.

Most of us can agree that our childhoods shaped our development and capability to function as an adult. But even the most successful adults can feel a sudden mood change of depression, anger, or irritability that comes from nowhere. What was the trigger that made this happen? Perhaps it was something you ate or someone you talked to. Maybe you were in an environment that triggered a feeling you could not understand, let alone plan for. All these factors surround us every day and essentially affect how healthily we are capable of living. The fittest person in the world, perhaps an Olympic athlete, will have an off day during a competition because of sudden, unexplained trigger in his or her environment or because his or her diet wasn't balanced for optimum performance. Whatever that trigger was, and triggers are different for everyone, it had such an impact that it may have caused that athlete to fail an Olympic event or, worse, cause a physical injury. Simply put, we all must come to understand what our personal mood triggers are, learn to overcome them, and make healthier choices in our lives. Once you are able to choose where you spend your time, with whom you share your life, and what food you consume, then you will gain positive control of how healthily you are able to physically live.

Preventive health starts with the food you choose to eat, right? Well, yes and no. There is no doubt that a diet rich in vegetables is more beneficial to a longer, healthier life, whereas eating animal food products (and French fries) will likely lead to adverse health problems. I know, French fries are awesome, and I personally would not want to live in a world without them. Inherently, it is worth your time to personally understand your body's ability to digest certain foods. For instance, it helps to keep a food journal for a period of time, perhaps thirty days or more, to identify how food (and alcohol and drugs) make you feel after it has been consumed. Specific food choices will be discussed in more detail later, but it is important to understand that food will absolutely alter your mood, which will then cause behaviors that may affect you and your family directly. Of course, we want our families to grow and develop both mentally and physically in the healthiest way possible. As parents, or even just food consumers in general, it starts with what we accept as food choices and how often we accept them.

In the United States, we are the top consumers of animal food sources and refined sugars, and we waste about 40 percent of all the food we buy per year (Gunders 2017). Can you imagine throwing away just under half of every meal you eat three times a day? We are also great at accepting donuts as a substantial breakfast choice for our children even though it does not have the basic nutrients needed for us to feel satiation. I mention children specifically here because we are in the midst of a child obesity epidemic in our country. Again, what the hell are we accepting as food choices? Ridiculous, you say? Well, a recent study released from the Cooper Institute and Dallas Independent School District confirms that "nearly 20 percent of school-aged children and 40 percent of adults are obese in the United States." Also, there is a clear link showing that children who maintained a healthier diet and were physically active for sixty minutes per day were, in fact, more successful as adults than children who did neither (Freeland 2019).

We all need food for survival, and we tend to forget about the quality level of food as we become consumed in our everyday lives. The quality of food determines how healthy we are, how long we live, and our ability to have the best lifestyle. Poor eating habits, likely developed from a triggered mood, are most commonly the culprit for weight gain, pain, and increased stress in our bodies and minds. Do you notice a cycle developing here?

Mood Trigger—Eating Habit—Overall Health Status

Let's break the cycle and give you some tools to work with. First, it is so important to truly understand your authentic self in terms of personal habits. Be humble and have humility to honestly identify shortfalls in your life that could cause any negative mood triggers or compulsive eating habits. Do not lie to yourself. Try to conceptualize how you feel about all things and people in your world. Then, at the very least, try to remember what you ate last and how that affected you hours and even days later. Journaling your food consumption for thirty days is a bit pretentious—I get it. But becoming more mindful of how food makes you feel will help motivate you to avoid certain foods altogether.

I will not only provide insight on my personal mood triggers and how to identify your own, but I will also provide simple guidelines to healthier food choices and healthier cooking techniques that are easy and realistic for busy households. As for expectation management from a reader's perspective, you will be able to relate with personal mood triggers and cook *real* whole-food meals that will set a positive mood, increase your energy, and prolong your quality of life. There are no recipes with processed foods included here, and I will primarily focus on increasing your vegetable consumption. Animal products and other fatty foods are relegated to side dishes, which I'll explain in more detail later. Also, refined sugars are intended to be consumed only occasionally, if at all. If you consume less sugary food than you already do now, I feel we made *some* progress toward a healthier diet. Above all, the main goal is to provide you with some tools to identify your mood triggers and inspire a healthier lifestyle, despite the odds against you!

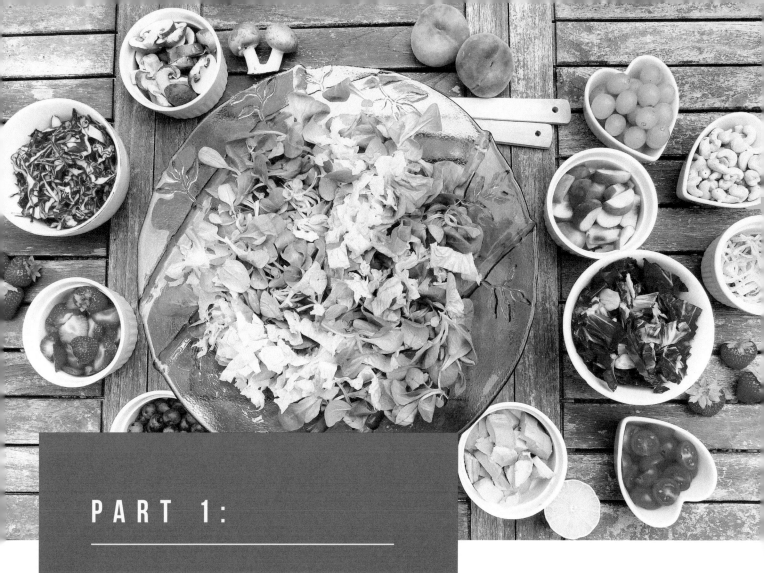

PART 1:

BALANCING YOUR HEALTH BEYOND THE PLATE

A healthy, balanced lifestyle means more than just eating vegetables and getting your daily workout done. Sure, this is a lifestyle book to increase your overall wellness within your busy life, but it is also important to understand that we are human beings and that life happens. Did you ever wake up late, grab a cup of coffee, and start the day completely off your game? Of course, we all have certain days in our lives when any stranger would judge us as a hot mess in passing. It's called life, and life happens—all the time. No one is living a perfectly uninterrupted life with an exact schedule, a healthy diet, and blissful thoughts every single day. But some of those stressful days could have been less hectic—or even avoided—with the right type of foods in our digestive systems, and a moment of meditation or physical activity wouldn't hurt either. But first, it's critical to understand that food is the foundation of our lives and literally sets us up for a mentally and physically healthier day. Essentially, what we habitually eat today will absolutely affect our overall health for the rest of our lives.

So, let's be real here for a second. It's Friday night, you are tired from a long week, and you order takeout from your favorite pizzeria or Thai restaurant. If it happens occasionally, you will not gain a ton of weight or notice your overall quality of health significantly diminish. If that were the case, there would not be a high demand for restaurants or other food businesses. You will, however, notice how you feel immediately after you eat that slice of heaven—your gut may feel bloated and uneasy or your energy level sluggish. Certain foods linger in our guts a bit longer than other types of food. It's just as well; everyone digests foods at a different rate entirely. So, while some may have to spend extra time taking care of business in the bathroom, others may not need a bathroom for days. Also, stomach sensitivity to processed foods, wheat, and dairy products, in particular, is getting more attention these days. We should not self-diagnose and claim that wheat products or gluten or dairy products are the culprits in poor digestive systems, weight gain, or adverse health effects. However, many people find digesting wheat and dairy products to be more difficult than digesting other foods. Personally, I feel an increase in energy and mentally more focused when I eat a diet rich in vegetables, fruits, seafood, nuts, and seeds. Refined sugars, specifically, need their very own section for discussion because of their negative health effects in our diets and in processed foods. Of course, sugar cannot be a controlled substance (or an illegal substance, for that matter) in our society, but becoming more mindful that sugar exists in our processed foods is a realistic approach. Who would ever want to miss out on eating a piece of birthday cake on that special day or an ice cream cone on the beach?

Not me. What it comes down to is that taking sugar completely out of your diet is not a realistic approach for living within our society. Well, at least not yet. Sugary treats should be something we look forward to on special occasions, all the while being mindful of the effects that sugar will have on us if we overconsume it too often.

The chapters in this book are aimed to give you a greater perspective on how and why your body craves certain foods and help you become more cognitive about how your body responds to food. I provide tips on how to become more mindful of your food habits and the environment in which you live. Although this is not written like a traditional cookbook, I also provide cooking methods for a typical household to guide you in making healthier meals. I give a few tips for better house party side dishes, meals for your family, and ways to keep the kids eating their vegetables. I share with you some of my personal compulsive eating and drinking habits, just to keep it classy. Seriously, though, I keep it real, and everything will absolutely relate to you in some way or another.

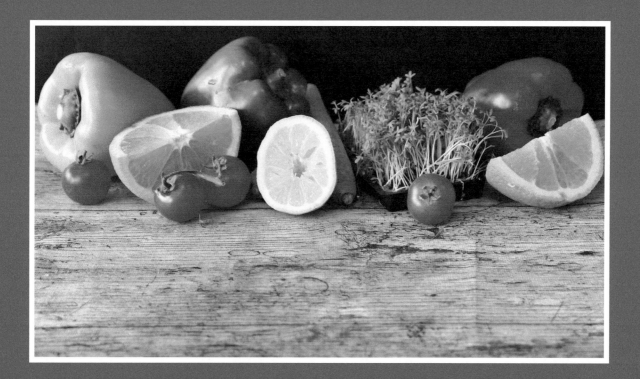

CHAPTER 1:

UNDERSTANDING MOOD TRIGGERS

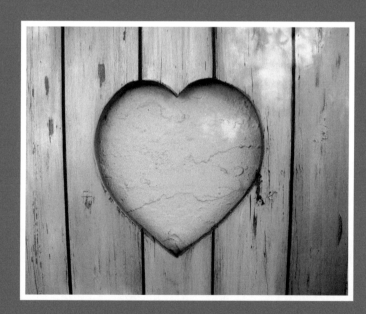

Stress consumes me. I ponder on uncertainties. I find temporary solutions in order to drive on. Breathe. Repeat. That is what I did for years until I had enough. And if you have ever survived or know someone who has survived a traumatic experience—an adverse childhood, a natural disaster, military combat, opioid addiction, alcoholism, domestic violence, mental health illness, divorced parents, death of a parent or loved one, cancer, or any illness you can possibly imagine—then you need to pay attention. You have developed some type of mood trigger that alters your ability to make simple decisions in your life. You may be walking obliviously in the grocery store on a typical food shopping excursion and then smell, see, or hear something that triggers a past detail in your life. Or maybe you attend a friendly get-together and are midway through a conversation when you remember a detail from your childhood. Maybe you hear a certain lyric or relatable phrase in a song playing on the radio. Next thing you know, you feel like absolute garbage, worthless, and ready to hide your face under a pillow. Something triggered your sudden and unexplained mood, and now your mind is left paralyzed to complete the simplest tasks. Something distracted you enough that you forgot why you even went upstairs or opened the refrigerator door. All you can do is stare at the wall and ask yourself, *What the hell did I come upstairs for again?* Something has blocked your ability to make that connection in your brain, and you are now distracted, frustrated, and ready to apply that coping mechanism—whatever that it is for you. Does this sound familiar?

After years of constantly battling distractions, I started to pay attention to certain things in my life. For instance, after a long run or intense cardio session in the gym, I was more focused on my daily tasks for the rest of the day. After doing something exciting enough that it initially caused butterflies in my stomach, I felt more confidence to try new things and meet new people. After hiking on a long trail to finally reach the mountain's summit, I felt accomplished and satisfied. Did I find my coping mechanism to deal with the stress and distractions? You bet I did. The physical activity that eventually evolved into a rigorous daily workout was my therapy to clear my head. To this day, I still look forward to an intense workout. The only problem is that those unexplained moods that seem to appear from nowhere never subsided. As a matter of fact, they showed up more often over time and eventually superseded the desire to move at all. Although it was hard to find motivation to function as an active person would, those distractions in my head grew louder over time. What is wrong with me? I really could not understand this new overwhelming feeling. I love all things active, all things happy, and all things that make people smile and laugh due to my canny, contagious character.

I was experiencing depression at the time, but I denied that depression was even a possibility. I am not normally a depressed person, and so I denied I needed support to work through these unexplainable feelings. "I am fine," I would say. *I just need a moment to vent to my friends or husband and speak what is on my mind out loud*, I would think. *I just need to push myself more in everything I do. More.* I thought the answer to dealing with depression was "more." It seems absurd now, but I really did put more on my plate—more distractions, more busy work, more of everything and anything to distract me from my own depression. I was literally working full time, taking college courses at night, flight lessons on weekends, and undergoing rigorous military training all simultaneously at one point - keeping busy to avoid dealing with my own emotions. It was a cycle. More busy work was followed by stress and then more depression. In the moment, I had no clue that I was depressed, let alone how to conceptualize dealing with it. This is where my support system needed to be locked in tight. A combination of venting to my husband and friends, the hard gym sessions, and plenty of alcohol was my coping mechanism for feeling like garbage - "my therapy," as I liked to call it. And as far I am concerned, all three coping mechanisms worked divinely for my mood at that point in time. Still, they did not solve the process of recurring moods, and I needed to find the trigger—or triggers—to get to the root of the problem. After having a chance to process and conceptualize these recurring moods, I realized that this shitty mood I kept feeling was my version of post-traumatic stress disorder, or PTSD.

In the Beginning

I met a guest speaker at a health summit while working toward my masters of public health and public health practice. He spoke of his past, and I was touched and amazed by his composure while telling his unbelievable story. He was a Hungarian-born Jewish survivor of the Holocaust, and the details were unimaginable; his spoken words gave me chills. His grandparents had been killed in Auschwitz when he was five months old, and he managed to escape the horror with his then-surviving, Nazi-enslaved relatives. To think about a five-month-old infant ripped away from the loving, warm, and nurturing arms of his family caused a tightness in my chest. I remember his story well, but his final talking points especially resonated with me. After describing the disturbing family tribulations forced upon him as an infant, he described the impact this particular experience had and has on him during his adult life.

I started to drift in my own thoughts as he was talking. I remember thinking, *I don't even remember my fifth birthday party or the first time I ever rode a bike, but I do clearly remember significant family disputes that will stay with me forever*. Looking back, *Jersey Shore* ratings could have dropped if some of my family disputes had been reality TV episodes. Nonetheless, I was maybe seven years old when I watched the domestic madness unravel in my backyard. The actual details of my parents' dispute are irrelevant, but that summer day is vividly committed to my memory. I can still see the lawn that needed to be cut, the partly clouded sky, and the red and white shed where we played bloody Mary for a good scare. Divorce can be an ugly experience, especially for a child exposed to entire childhood of domestic violence, but my life seemed to be petty nonsense at this point. But was it?

The speaker continued telling his story, as well as others with similar traumatic childhood experiences, and described the linkage to their particular addictions that developed over time, such as drug and alcohol abuse, chronic disease, and poor behavioral habits. He went on to ask the audience whether the actual substance itself was the root of the problem or something or someone caused them to deal with an underlying problem that, in so doing, resulted in substance abuse. I found myself immediately defensive, as I have always thought that substance abuse was connected to a development of a disease in the sense of a particular abnormal condition that negatively affects the structure of function of our brain. Now, I began to understand it from a different angle.

I kept listening to his remarkable story, and the details of his particular childhood experience brought tears to my eyes. Everyone can relate in some capacity to incidences within their own childhood. Their own situations may not be as horrific as the Holocaust, but everyone has had some direct or indirect childhood experience that impacted them in some way, even if it is just that you happened to find yourself with your kids in the grocery store and witnessed strangers having some sort of a verbal or physical dispute. Our children are taking permanent, mental notes. They are developing blueprints of their lives as we allow them to see, hear, and feel exposures of all types. I heavily question the long-term effects on children of verbal and physical abuse from their parents. Often times we forget that verbal abuse can be the most common form of unreported abuse. I have personally witnessed incidents where parents verbally express that their child's existence in life was a ploy to save their marriage. It sounds as harsh as it felt for that child who was left feeling empty, worthless, and unwanted in this world. I can only imagine how the mood triggers from this repetitive incident alone will play out when this particular child reaches adulthood.

Within my own childhood experiences, I learned there is so much more that augments the undeniable truth of one's authentic self. That is, we all deal with our life experiences in such diverse ways that there can be no formula, medication, or educated [professional] answers to explain why we as humans behave a certain way. It is expected that adverse childhood experiences will tally up during an ugly divorce, for example. In the same breath, every person should spend the time processing their own childhood experiences and perhaps identify and understand their own mood triggers. I have actually spent years doing just this, and I will tell you there is a clear, defined linkage between my childhood and the moods I have as an adult. I can predict when I will be irritable, at the very least, and catch myself before snapping back at my children. My siblings, on the other hand, have an entirely different story to tell.

Let's just say, for example, you lost a parent early on in your childhood due to combat, addiction, or other related health issues. Perhaps you grew up with a relative who had a drug or alcohol addiction, and it was common to witness the culminating result of rock bottom for that person in your life. Perhaps your parents were not exactly Ward and June Cleaver from the 1957 TV series *Leave It to Beaver* and your normal childhood consisted of dysfunctional parents who literally never demonstrated love for each other, compassion for raising children, or even a cordial moment between them. Maybe you grew up in a household where alcohol, drugs and domestic violence were the normal after-school special, rather than participating in school sports, clubs or other activities. If you can relate to any of these examples, you developed some sort of mood trigger during your childhood. And I just listed a few common ACEs. The fact that ACEs are a difficult topic to study was the top motivator to add this personal segment to this book. I absolutely believe that mood triggers exist and are clearly associated with our past childhood experiences. What is intriguing is the fact that siblings may experience the same childhood exposures yet live very different lives as adults. An inauspicious parenting style, at the very least, is sure to reveal expected adverse childhood experiences, as most people would agree. I, however, eventually learned to accept my parents' need to separate from each other and understand their personal characteristics early on in my adult life. More importantly, it wasn't until recently that I accepted that I cannot change them and need to love them unconditionally, without judgment, just as they love me in their own unique way. It is difficult for most people to conceptualize that we are in control of nothing except our own behaviors and actions. Regardless of what type of hand we were dealt as children, we can always choose our own environment, food choices, and social activities. We can always try to influence others to lead a healthier and more fulfilling life. In any case, I try to lead by example for my own children knowing the significant impact I will have in *their* adult life. To this day, I try to live by a set of values that resonates closely with this in mind, especially when dealing with family matters. Our children are watching us and developing their own set of values. We cannot screw this up. We cannot accept adversity into their lives and if adverse exposures are present in your child's life, talk to them about the situation in detail. Communicate effectively. Help them process the situation and learn from it, then enable them to grow into a better person from there.

As my personal story with understanding mood triggers unfolded, I realized there must be people out there who can relate and need to know that they are not alone. Case in point, I can keenly remember being pregnant in Alaska with my daughter and learning that my distant loved ones were dealing with a downward spiraling cycle of a ten-plus-year opioid addiction. The type of household that my niece and nephew were raised in was left to my imagination. I learned that, by ages five and nine, they had already been exposed to counts of domestic violence, parents who were physically abusive to each other, substance abuse, psychological and verbal abuse, one parent with multiple incarcerations, and situations only they would be able to describe. Tears fill my eyes as I write this personal segment because I felt vulnerable in a way that I had never felt before. I could not help the situation, and I blamed myself since I spent twelve years away from them while serving in the army. I blamed myself for placing my career ahead of my loved ones and blindly heard the aftermath of arrests and disputes from afar. After serving three combat deployments and then transitioning to civilian life, I felt like the once-expected PTSD during this reintegration period was a full-on tsunami of emotions.

During my combat experiences and exposures, I did not come into contact with enemy firearms very often. That is not exactly how our current warfare is strategically designed these days. However, I did endure real sacrifices and feelings of my life being uncertain often enough to vividly remember intense situations that will haunt me for a lifetime. If you served in the military and were ever deployed into combat, you know exactly what I am talking about. For my nonmilitary readers, imagine a foreign place in southwest Asia, a camp-like base setting with uniform, small, aluminum buildings (or combat housing units) and all the details Hollywood likes to portray for you— you know, camouflage uniforms, desert-painted up-armored vehicles, tents lined up in rows, and plenty of dust in the air. I have many combat incidents that are clearly played over and over again in my head, but one in particular is relevant to mention here. As I remember, I walked back to my housing unit after a shower and stopped to talk to friend who knew my husband (thank God) when a few rocket-propelled grenades (RPGs) suddenly starting breaching our forward operating base. The housing unit that I was originally headed to had a nearby building destroyed by the RPG. I was twenty-five feet from the crossfire at the time. I knew and worked with the soldier who was killed that day while sleeping a few units down from mine during this incident. This is just one example of the many close-call incidents I experienced during my military deployments. This was one life lost due to a combat-related incident that would be only the first of many more fallen comrades I knew and worked with. I took every American death very personally, felt an intense need for revenge, and never really learned to process these emotions properly, if ever.

These types of incidents stay with you for a lifetime, and they need to be mentally processed to move forward. Because I had these experiences, I understand my own father, a Vietnam veteran, much better now, and his later life decisions correlate with PTSD most accurately. During the Vietnam era, I can only imagine that no one really understood why my father had sporadic moods and irritable moments, as miscommunication with family members was a common result. Just think about it—my father departed from his one-year Vietnam tour to head back to his family with a bus ticket and a toothbrush in his hand, for God's sake. There was no mandatory mental health evaluation or reintegration period. There was no time to mentally process what had happened in Vietnam, and no one could possibly empathize with him at the time or even to this day perhaps. This is a perfect example of a major factor that could weigh heavily on your marriage and your children later on in life. I have a better relationship with my father today because I understand the mood trigger concept developed from past incidents and traumatic experiences. My grandfather, a World War II veteran, must have endured similar effects of what we define today as PTSD during *his* reintegration process as well. And just as expected, I can easily identify and understand where there is a disconnection among family members alike. Three generations of combat veterans each with very different experiences, yet we all developed some type of mood trigger that correlates with irritability, stress and depression.

Every veteran will hold significant war demons deep inside his or her head, and healing depends on many personal variables. Therefore, it is only right to state that my combat experiences cannot be compared to those of any other veteran anywhere in this world. However, it is important to acknowledge that combat exposures will leave everyone with mood triggers that may be difficult for family members to comprehend in its entirety. For me, I worked through my adverse experiences in silence. I kept most fears and uncertainties to myself. I learned to adapt to combat experiences fairly quickly because I understood survival in the sense that my childhood shaped that Viking mentality I mentioned before. I was comfortable with the risks associated with serving my country. It is almost paradoxical to associate post-combat experiences with my childhood, but it makes perfect sense in terms of the decisions I have made in my adult life. Essentially, survival mode was my norm.

I do believe that my childhood experiences literally shaped me into the person I am today, but how we deal with our past misfortune as adults is something we still have control of. For instance, I resorted to intense gym sessions and alcohol binge-drinking as my outlet, or coping mechanism, as research would have predicted. Today, about twenty-two veterans take their lives every day due to post-traumatic stress disorder (PTSD) inflicted by decades of combating terror (Johnson 2019). Moreover, researchers are overwhelmed with information to adequately study combat-related experiences and horrific shootings in our own homeland that seem to happen on a weekly, if not daily, basis. The aftermath of trauma both overseas and at home affects everyone. These experiences affect our moods, our eating habits, and our ability to essentially live a healthy life.

I could very easily have become part of this very statistic. Instead, I felt that suicide was a weak-minded option, and I constantly felt empowered by being able to make my situation better. It was my niche and probably still is. That is, I am addicted to making something out of nothing. I am addicted to feeling confident, successful, and well-balanced as an individual, yet humbly understanding and accepting that humans are imperfect and I am no exception. The army lesson I learned that perhaps resonates with me best is, *always leave something (or a place) better than you found it*. It affects everything I do, and I am addicted to the reaction from people when they see a turd really can be polished, so to speak.

With the current opioid epidemic on the rise and children being in the mix of it all, the adverse cycle is most likely to continue. I like to believe that doctors who have the ability to prescribe drugs to their patients are exhausting all other means of holistic approaches to healing, rather than resorting to a pharmaceutical quick fix. Regarding doctors prescribing medication, I heard a colleague once say, "They don't want to completely cure you, but they don't want you to die either." The common question I ask myself is, "Are medical professionals running a profitable business, or are they genuinely providing health care to their patients?" Interestingly enough, those in the medical profession as are asking the same questions and widely choosing the latter.

I work to think optimistically as childhood exposures is an extremely broad topic. My thoughts raced on the word *exposure* as most people automatically associate the word with something negative, such as physical, sexual, or emotional abuses; neglect; domestic violence; substance misuse within a household; parental separation or divorce; or an incarcerated parent. The list of negative exposures can be as colorful and exhausting as your mind allows. I like to believe that positive exposures can erase the negative effects that adverse experiences may have had on a child. I am hopeful that evidence-based education on the reversal of negative experiences during early-childhood brain development will be required in academia. I hope that parents will become educated on ACEs and PTSD and understand the positive effects that love and affection will have on our children. Love is very powerful, and kids need a lot of it. I try to do my best to stop what I am doing when my daughter needs help putting shoes on her baby doll or when my son wants to show me his version of the ABCs by using an entire sheet of stickers on our dog. Sure, I really want to say, "Hang on, honey, I am in the middle of something" or lash out verbally and say, "What the hell are you doing to the dog?" But honestly, what could be more important than your children's need for a parent to pay attention to them? To educate them? To be the example for them? Our actions speak volumes, and our children are taking mental notes on everything we do. I am ironically grateful for the childhood experiences my divorced parents gave me because they conditioned me to excel in the military as an effective leader. That Viking mentality gave me the strength and drive to move forward through adverse experiences, learn from them, and apply those lessons in my adult life.

In terms of depression and understanding my mood triggers, I realized that I tried to change my parents' relationship, or lack thereof, through my personal successes. Military, college, promotions, awards, achievements—the hard work was all worth it only if there was a proud parent to show for it. And they were very proud, but that did not change their focus on their disdain for each other. Mistakenly, I took it personally, and eventually, after what I thought were years of disappointment, my emotions became numb and callused over. Unfortunately, even though I understand the impact that divorce had on my childhood, those years of disappointment are enough to trigger a mood even today—an irritable, worthless, and then depressed kind of mood. Intuitively, I will find disappointment with either parent and almost immediately become irritable enough to snap at my children, feel anxiety, or reach for a stiff drink. The army provided a promising organization after years of disappointment, and I embraced serving long-term with open arms. Back then it was 1997 when I enlisted myself to escape what my childhood may have predicted for my adult life. Ironically, I thought giving myself to a higher purpose was the answer to solve my issues at home. Knowing now what the army did for my well-being, I would still make that career decision again. In the end, my drive for independent success defines who I am today most accurately.

So Now What?

The most common predicted outcomes for ACEs and PTSD are nothing short of addiction, eating disorders, heart disease, anxiety, and other chronic diseases. The list goes on, but it is probably one of the most difficult studies of our time since we are talking about how we feel about people we love. Perhaps, success could be a possible outcome for those who live with ACEs or PTSD if a healthier path was an option. Comparing one's experiences to those of another is not the intent here, but it is so important to reflect on your personal childhood exposures and pay attention to your mood triggers. For me, as soon as I remembered a childhood memory, I would feel irritable with a heavy sense of worthlessness. Eventually, I grew to understand that my depressed state of mind stemmed from a few major exposures that occurred from infancy to seventeen years old, and then I joined the army. Essentially, by enlisting, I already changed what may have been statistically predicted for me. It wasn't until a few years ago that I realized how severe my own PTSD was at that very moment. I was so concerned about family members' being in the middle of an opioid-infused crisis that I never gave myself time to mentally transition from twelve years of military service to a functioning civilian, let alone process the combat exposures, hardships, and sacrifices that service members endure but rarely discuss in an open forum.

As soon as I was reminded of these experiences, I immediately felt a sense of worthlessness and a need for self-destruction that literally left me mentally paralyzed. I found myself with no drive or will to function in society more often than not. I stopped caring about my personal fitness goals, and at the time, nutrition was defined as gin and tonic. And when I was not drinking to numb the feelings of worthlessness, I kept my schedule somewhat neurotically busy. My husband and friends would often pull me out of my funk just by a simple call or reminder that I was not alone.

The mood triggers were sporadic. Considering my role as a leader at the time, I shunned the idea of starting a mental health record. I thought it was best to turn to Catholicism to help fight my demons in secret. It was a common and unspoken path for some service members. "Go see the chaplain," was the guidance often recommended to our soldiers. And so, I did. I received my communion and was confirmed into the Catholic Church as an adult in the process of my reintegration from my second combat tour. My record was unscathed, and I marched on. I continued my career and was off to my third deployment shortly after without any delay. I am raising my children as Catholics today, and I have no regrets for the path I chose; however, mental health counseling from a professional counselor could have expedited the healing process.

Mental health counseling is probably the most important support system for service members since our nation's first conflict, yet PTSD is just now gaining more attention than ever before. I was too concerned about my military record having a slight trace of "she is crazy" written in it, and rightfully so; that may have been the case at the time, unfortunately. Today, the military has taken responsibility for the previous PTSD shortcomings for our post-deployment service members in support of the reintegration process. Two decades of war and conflict are overwhelming for any organization, and supporting each service member adequately throughout them is more so. With that being said, there is no shame in identifying your own personal mood triggers and being humble enough to make an appointment. To my veteran readers, or anyone suffering from depression, taking that first step could absolutely save your life. This had such an impact in my life that I chose to go back to college and find a way to help other people figure their shit out. Just as well—I was in need of a fresh beginning.

After my military career, I aspired to be a competitive CrossFit athlete and completed my master's in public health and public health practice on my best days. On other days, my mind was on a roller coaster of emotions. The combination of numerous domestic disputes that were close to home and the constant haunting of Iraq and Afghanistan were peaking and seemed endless. It was then that I started to really pay attention to my moods and then connecting certain interactions with family members and combat-related incidents. Depression was expected after being reminded of these negative thoughts. My eating was less than subpar at best or was not a priority at all. I looked sickly and skinny. I was vulnerable for the first time in my life because I actually felt some sort of emotion I could not explain—I felt absolutely vulnerable. Vulnerability was exactly what I needed to finally let go of decades of adverse experiences and figure out how to really enjoy life again.

I was feeling my best when I was surrounded by a community of supportive, physically active people and simultaneously eating a healthier diet. The combination of these two factors was the key to finally resolving the uncontrollable mood triggers developed over time from ACEs and PTSD. I was happy, socially engaged, and exceeding my body's abilities and expectations regularly. It was my mental therapy that I so desperately needed. I was not new to the health and fitness lifestyle.

I had always been athletic, competitive, and willing to optimistically be the fun energy in any room with any crowd. At this point, my life was on the upswing because I had started to become mentally and emotionally healthy instead of emotionally numb. I started to truly understand that food and mindfulness were just as important as my physically capabilities. I started to focus on mentally processing the adversity in my past and dedicating my time to changing things in my life I actually had control of—food, exercise, and my social environment. Essentially, feeling healthy is a balance of a healthy diet, daily exercise, and the social environment. Once I started to really hone in on food and exercise, I even slept better as well.

Being able to first understand my mood triggers, accept them, and face them with courage was imperative. My husband stood by me through the thick of it. Our ability to communicate at this point in our marriage is counter to the statistics and expectations of people we knew. We were a dual-military couple with multiple deployments, combat exposures, adverse childhood experiences from both sides of the spectrum, and years of poor eating and drinking habits, and still we beat the odds. We became mentally stronger during this period in our relationship, and my daughter is proof of that. I started to get my shit together, take back my life, and push on the way I knew. I let go of uncertainties I had no control over and could not change. I started to become grateful that I had survived my military experiences and cherished the strong people I had met throughout my career. I started to truly understand family values and how to love my husband and children unconditionally.

As a result of understanding my mood triggers, I accept my family for who they are, and I am wholeheartedly committed to showing my children what a loving home feels like. I purposely show my husband affection in front of my children to demonstrate how loving parents share their lives together, just as a loving and nurturing home also involves providing healthy meals and a safe environment for proper brain development and growth throughout adolescence. Everyone's life story is unique, and everyone will have different mood triggers that lead to different eating habits or, worse, addictions. It is so important to be true to yourself and take the time to identify your mood triggers. Understand that you are enough in this world and that doing more has the potential to exacerbate stress and depression. Make it a priority to change your social or physical environment and diet if, in fact, your moods are causing adversity in your life. Your behavioral habits will eventually morph into a lifestyle of which you could potentially lose control of, a lifestyle that may preclude your ability to be the best person you can possibly be mentally, physically, and socially.

Embrace the Suck and Drive On

By now you have read a few personal examples that hopefully gave you something to think about. Everyone has some sort of past that shaped his or her well-being and ultimately influenced decisions in his or her life. Some people do not have all the answers right now as to why they suddenly feel a certain way. Some may not even know what they were exposed to as children and need to do some personal digging. Some may be in the midst of a stressful lifestyle and have not even determined that poor eating habits are prevalent and depression is creeping up.

If you can resonate with any of these mood trigger topics that I have mentioned so far or know someone who can, then it is imperative that you take some time for self-reflection. Take action and talk to someone—anyone. Take the time to analyze your childhood, your personal experiences, and any traumatic events that took place in your life. You owe it to yourself to process the emotional connection with others and get yourself mentally right again. You owe it to your family to work through misplaced mood swings, identify the triggers, and handle them with confidence. You owe it to yourself and your health.

Whether counseling with a professional psychotherapist, a licensed social worker, or a friend, or even a private prayer with God, there is always some support system that can assist you in identifying your mood triggers. Ask questions with someone you trust, and I bet that person will raise a red flag and point you in the right direction. No shame. No guilt. No regrets. It is critical that you communicate to your loved ones clearly in order to help you process the adversity that may be causing a coping mechanism to persist, like abusing alcohol or drugs or stress eating, for example. And remember, there is no shame in identifying a mood trigger and dealing with it. When you do, you will naturally develop your own expectation management on how to handle your moods and continue on in your life with confidence. Simply, it is not just "embracing the suck" of stress and depression; rather, it is more important to honestly "understand the suck" and learn how to drive on.

CHAPTER 2:

ADVERSE CHILDHOOD EXPERIENCES (ACES), POST-TRAUMATIC STRESS DISORDER (PTSD), AND HEALTHY FOOD CHOICES

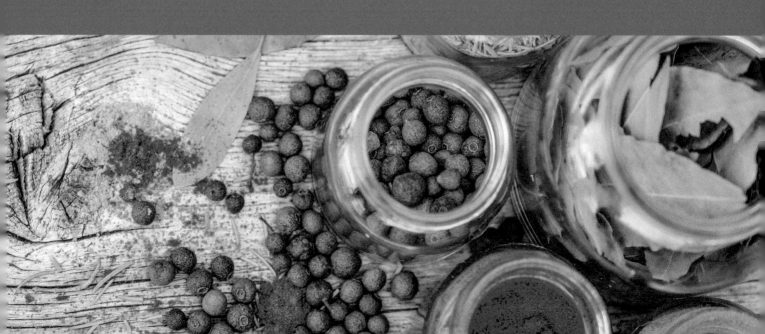

I explained that it is possible that mood triggers developed during our childhoods and are difficult to understand in their entirety. I discussed that mood triggers have the potential to cause poor health behaviors and potentially obscure our ability to make sound decisions regarding what we accept as food. I discussed that significant, adverse experiences of fear and uncertainty are, in fact, known to be connected to developing stress, irritability, depression, and adverse health outcomes. What I have not mentioned is that all these experiences, from either from ACEs or PTSD-causing incidents, continue to disrupt the connection from our brains to our bodies. Even though a particular incident may have happened years ago, it is likely that the physiological functioning in the brain centers and neurotransmitter systems have been damaged in such a way that logical connections are disrupted (American Academy of Pediatrics 2014). Those compulsive eating sessions we have are likely the result of this disconnection—we may have a broken circuit, if you will. As you can imagine, eating a massive amount of sugar-based foods or drinking a bottle of wine every day is not only damaging to our digestive systems, it can also lead to heart disease, high-blood pressure, type-2 diabetes, and other chronic illnesses. Over time, these destructive eating habits also establish a mental pattern that our bodies respond to. Our brains eventually start to recognize a familiar moment of stress and depression, and in response, we grab our favorite go-to comfort food in an effort to divert those negative feelings. Our brains and bodies have now become comfortable with the notion of temporary satisfaction, and we literally begin to crave that temporary fix. Whether it is a specific comfort food, alcohol, or drug of choice, the feelings of stress, irritability, or depression are delayed for the moment. Those compulsive sessions of eating and substance abuse are likely due to our personal ways of mentally processing stress or depression, and we all have become great at rationalizing why we do it.

Rationalizing Food Choices

Rationalizing what we accept for food choices is done completely on a personal level. Eating patterns are, essentially, a physiological collaboration between our brains and our bodies. We all handle stress eating differently; if you are like me, you stop eating altogether. We all rationalize eating habits in one form or another in order to give ourselves permission to literally eat whatever we want whenever we want. Somewhere along in our lives, we decided that certain foods are acceptable to consume at a relentless rate. Take dark chocolate-covered almonds, for example.

Did you ever find yourself having a bad day, nervous about something, or pondering something in your mind? Suddenly it is okay to consume an entire bag of those sweet, delicious morsels in under five minutes. And when someone questions you on your human vacuum-like capabilities, you simply explain that dark chocolate is better than milk chocolate, almonds are actually healthy for you, and the excuses are endless. The fact that you ignored the sugar content entirely and the number of calories per serving was never considered are irrelevant. My husband admits to rationalizing his obsession with eating Doritos. In his words, "As a kid I often ate entire bag of Doritos in one sitting, and I still crave them today." So, is it okay to continue eating an entire bag of Doritos because you did that when you were a kid? Of course not. Perhaps you are not a stress eater but absolutely have no problem rationalizing excessive drinking. I'm guilty of pouring an adult beverage anytime I feel a bit stressed. I literally just caught myself telling my friends that I am a better parent after a few glasses of wine. Sure, all little tykes are expected to test their parents' patience every now and then, but I noticed I am an incredibly irritable parent on days I skipped the gym, drank too much coffee, and forgot to eat something substantial all day. It may be logical to stop for a moment, eat a nutrient-rich meal, and drink a glass of water, but wine always wins over common sense for me. I believe the typical daily sequence of events starts when it is the witching hour in our household—about five o'clock in the evening. The noise level rises, the news program on the television is louder than my stovetop fan, and I am telling my children, "You are driving me crazy" as I pour my first glass of wine for the night. What is worse is the fact that my wine drinking continues all night, and in the morning—you guessed it—I am even more irritable when I try to wake up. These are both classic cases of rationalizing food choices all while subconsciously overconsuming calories, or adult beverages in my case. Rationalizing stress eating (or drinking alcohol) is an act of lying to yourself. And most would agree that we are completely aware that this is a destructive lifestyle, yet we continue to do it.

Rationalizing our food choices most likely originated in our childhoods, in terms of the household environment. That is, how we were raised and, for some of us, the aftermath of survival mode living with ACEs and PTSD may have caused specific eating patterns. I recall many intense dinner moments during my childhood that could be compared to riding the *Zipper*, a type of carnival ride, at our local county fair. Why? Well, I never knew what to expect each night while eating dinner at my house. I was always a ball of nerves and on the verge of puking. The environment put me on edge because of the constant uncertainty of family members at the table, and I had a strong sense that I needed to rush through my meal and get the hell out of dodge. Animosity was a common feeling in our household, and it was always best to eat and move out as quickly as possible. Ironically, this eat-and-go mentality was again introduced into my life when I attended basic training in the military. Although I understood the reason that eating was so rushed then, I still find myself in a hurry to finish my meal more often than not today. Now, as I watch my children grow up, I try to eat slower with them, actually enjoy the taste if my food, and appreciate the conservation and quality family time at the dinner table. I challenge you to do the same. Slow down a bit during your meals and actually enjoy the flavor of your food choice and the company you choose to eat with. Eating more slowly enables your food to properly digest and satisfies your appetite. It also enables you to be completely mindful of the amount of food you are consuming all while establishing positive memories of the eating event itself.

Even if you are committed to eating slower, certain go-to food choices are a product of our particular childhood environments. For instance, ketchup, or any condiment for that matter, has the potential to make it into every meal we eat. The most common table condiment you will find in a restaurant is ketchup, right next to the salt, pepper, and packets of sugar. Ketchup, mayonnaise, mustard, hot sauce, whatever you can think of—our society has taught us that we need to add flavor to our meals. I admit to establishing an obsession with Tabasco sauce on my fried eggs, for example. What we tend to forget is that our favorite condiment also has additional calories and a ton of preservatives most of us cannot even pronounce. Additionally, the second ingredient in ketchup will most likely be sugar. I like to believe that if food was seasoned right during the cooking process, additional condiments are unnecessary. There is no reason to dip our fries in some type of processed sauce or condiment to make them taste good. Rather, cut fresh sweet potatoes into wedges, coat them with olive oil and seasoning, and then bake them until crispy. The flavor is amazing, and it is a better choice of a vegetable overall. Once I started cooking healthier meals, I realized that seasoning food properly helped me avoid adding processed sauces and condiments into my diet. Using more spices, herbs, seasoning, and fresh ingredients is not only a healthier choice, it is the most flavorful choice as well.

Why Healthy Food Choices Matter

Making subtle changes for a healthier lifestyle can be intimidating at first. Some eating patterns are embedded so deeply in our roots that we cannot fathom another way of surviving, let alone becoming mindful to toxic food choices. Some of us were raised on fast food and never really gave the health impacts of this diet much thought. It is no secret that Americans are the top consumers of fast foods, with burgers being the most popular item on the menu. Likewise, it should be no surprise that the prevalence of obesity in America is reported to be 18.5% and affects about 13.7 million children and adolescents (CDC 2018). With these numbers on the rise, it is important to choose healthier food options for our children, especially as the socioeconomic gap continues to widen. Fundamentally, parents provide the example for their children, and so we need to communicate the value of healthier food choices and portions to them. As a child, I recall the days of not being excused from the dinner table until my plate was completely cleared off. Eating dinner was practically involuntary and done under duress work if veal was served for dinner. Nonetheless, everything had to be eaten. Nowadays, I tend to forget that my three-year-old has a stomach half the size of mine. I constantly try to feed my kids more food than they actually need, and I am ultimately annoyed when they waste food. Proportional food choices are something I need to work on as well.

Healthier food choices will make a positive difference in terms of addressing the long-term effects of ACEs and PTSD. It is critical to conceptualize that the effects of stress and depression are exacerbated by a poor diet or alcohol consumption. Fast-food choices are generally going to augment emotional setbacks because of how you will feel after eating processed foods. Also, eating poorly will cause internal physical stress on your digestive system, all while your irritable mood is well underway. Stress and depression will eventually overcome your ability or desire to complete the simplest of tasks. On the other hand, healthier food choices provide you with nutrient-rich calories that allow you to function more efficiently, both physically and mentally. Eating a diet that is primarily plant-based will physically support digestion more effectively, mentally provide you with the ability to focus better, and emotionally give you the confidence to face your fears and deal with problems. How can a healthy diet do all that? Well, if your brain and stomach are satisfied with the nutrients they receive, they can focus on other things like producing energy. Otherwise, if you short-change your nutrition, miscommunication will occur between your brain and, essentially, the rest of your body. That miscommunication causes you to feel anxiety and even more stress. There are some types of positive stress factors, such as starting a new job, moving to new location or, perhaps, you decided to undergo some type training or higher education. Positive stress helps you grow as an individual and can be exciting to feel this type of stress – leaving you feeling uplifted and confident. That miscommunication between your brain and stomach, on the other hand, that potentially causes you to feel anxiety and stress can easily end up as a period of depression. Negative stress factors are likely to lead you to a state of depression and will inevitably cause poor eating habits. When I start feeling a wave of stress and depression that originated from my ACEs and PTSD, I have learned to take a deep breath and except that I need to humbly control my emotions. Then, I communicate with my husband that I need a moment to myself to drink water and burn a few calories off in the gym. Literally, ten to twenty minutes of resetting my mind will get me back on track. Replenishing the calories that I burned off with an apple or banana and drinking water (yes, simple water) helps my brain refocus and appease my stomach until dinner is ready. All of this would not be easy without my husband's support; effective communication with loved ones goes a long way. Essentially, breaking the cycle on depression is nearly impossible without human support. No one is immune to feeling some degree of depression at some point in their life – that should be expected. What is critical is how we deal with depression when it is prevalent in our lives.

CHAPTER 3:

MAKE IT YOUR PERSONAL CHOICE

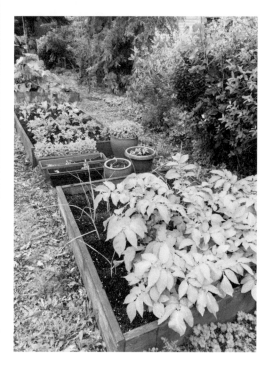

Just as eating comfort foods is something we commonly rationalize in order to temporarily satisfy our emotions, it only makes sense to identify and change certain eating habits that enhance these mood swings. There is no doubt that Americans consume way too much sugar within our trending diets. It is critical to understand that sugar addiction is a biological disorder that is driven by hormones and neurotransmitters that control sugar and carbohydrate cravings. As a result, we overeat more often than not. In this chapter, I will provide simple solutions to increase real, whole foods in your diet, stabilize blood sugar levels by eating more healthy protein and carbohydrate choices, decrease sugar consumption entirely, and reduce stress. It is critical to acknowledge that eating healthfully and living a balanced lifestyle will have long-term effects on your body's chemistry and overall wellness. However, you have to make the personal choice to commit to making a healthier lifestyle. I will explain how to do it simply through food choices in this chapter.

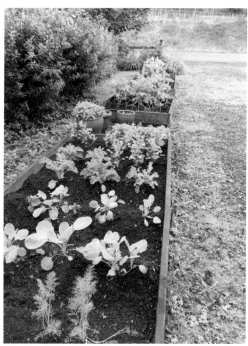

Consider adopting these three simple food guidelines to kick start a healthier diet.

- Plant-based, whole foods are always the way to go as it just makes sense to eat real food. Always try to eat plant-based foods in their rawest form. Challenge yourself to stay away from all processed foods, to include animal products.

- Shop in the produce aisle as much as possible. Eat organic, grass-fed animal products if you absolutely have to include animal products in your diet. Always be aware of the processing that took place prior to buying your meats, poultry, and fish as it is expected that hormones, preservatives, and other ingredients were added.

- Fresh vegetables and fruits always taste better, but never rule out frozen vegetables and fruits in order to make your budget work for you. The nutritional benefits of fresh verses frozen are the same.

Eating Local Produce

Organic gardening will always guarantee fresh produce and self-gratification of a healthier lifestyle, but not everyone has a green thumb. Have no worries because farmers' markets are a win-win! At a local market, you will find the freshest produce that tastes the best and supports your local agriculture productions at the same time. Buying local is great way to alleviate the processing time otherwise needed for vegetables and fruit to make it to your table, as well as to completely avoid adding excessive packaging materials into our landfills. Everyone wins if you are buying local produce.

Unfortunately, seasonal production and cost may deter you from buying your goods from a local vendor and encourage you to shop at a commercially stocked grocery store. If this is the case, always be mindful of where the goods are coming from and think about the processing and travel time it took for anything to make it to your community. For example, transporting avocados from Mexico to Alaska may take several weeks and pose a risk of numerous environmental exposures (e.g., temperature, humidity, ventilation, biotic activity, gases, toxicity, contamination, insects, feces, etc.). Not to mention that imported goods cost more. A lot more. For instance, I will have to pay at least $3.50 for one very ripe (if not rotten) avocado because I live in rural Alaska. Solution, I try to eat locally grown foods as much as possible.

The Dirty Truth on Sugar

If I could encourage you to make one healthy change from reading this book, it would be to limit your daily sugar consumption. It is the very least you can do help prolong a healthier lifestyle, but it's not easy. There is a very good reason there are compelling parallels between the American diet and the obesity epidemic. And to our dismay, it is not entirely our fault. Processed food is produced in such a way that a sugar ingredient always makes its way into the most basic food options on the shelf. Seriously, there are at least sixty-one different names for sugar that are listed on food labels. Some may sound familiar to you, such as sucrose, high-sucrose corn syrup, barley malt, dextrose, maltose, and rice syrup, to name a few. Dr. Joseph M. Mercola published a study finding that more than 50 percent of all Americans consume one half pound of sugar *per day* (Mercola 2010). That is over 180 pounds of sugar per year! There are too many preventive health problems that derive from a high-sugar diet to mention in just one chapter of this book. However, the underlying truth about sugar is that excessive consumption may be the largest factor causing obesity and chronic disease in our country. Depression is a type of chronic disease. It is a state of low mood and aversion to activity, which can affect a person's thoughts, behavior, tendencies, feelings, and sense of well-being. The Centers of Disease Control and Prevention reports that "one

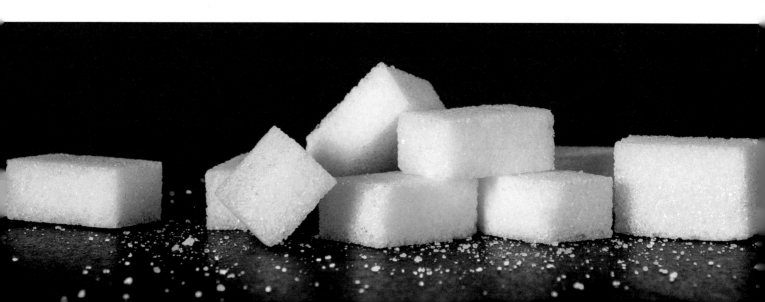

out of every six adults will have depression… and affects about 16 million American adults every year" (CDC 2018). Hence, sugar should be treated as a recreational drug. Ridiculous, you say?

Well, sugar is addictive, and your brain responds to it by releasing opioids and dopamine, thus causing addiction-like behavior. A sugar-dependence is easily developed over a short period of time, and behaviors can be closely related to neurochemical changes in the brain that are identical to changes that occur with addictive drugs. Your body can also build up a tolerance to sugar in such a way that it alters your craving, hunger, and satiety. The damage sugar does to your metabolism and liver, for example, is just one profoundly significant result without the buzz of recreational drugs or alcohol. What is the fun in that?

Evidence suggests that high-sugar diets will mostly likely lead to obesity, inflammation, and high triglyceride, blood sugar, and blood pressure levels, all of which are risk factors for heart disease. Diabetes is also a result of prolonged high-sugar consumption that in time drives resistance to insulin, a hormone produced by the pancreas that regulates blood sugar levels. Cancer, acne, depression, high cholesterol, skin aging, cellular aging, decreased energy, and fatty liver are other side effects from high doses of sugar. And, the worse part, our children are the forerunners of the commercialized sugar market and the youngest to join the obesity epidemic (CDC 2016).

Seriously, a moment on the lips causes a lifetime on the hips. I know, it is cliché to put it in these terms, but it really does make sense to think of it like this. What would life be like without a sweet treat to look forward to every now and then? Why is something so simple so terrible for you? Besides all the known health risks associated with sugar, it is critical to give yourself an honest evaluation of your personal sugar consumption. This requires some time spent on reading labels and being completely mindful of your daily intake. To my coffee drinkers, I am sorry to tell you that you may be setting yourself up for failure the moment you add your favorite vanilla or hazelnut creamer to your cup of joe. Try to drink black coffee or switch to tea if you can stand it. Caffeinated beverages are meant to wake you up, right? So why drink a beverage with added sugar that will drain your energy moments later? And don't be fooled by the sugar-free marketing campaigns. Remember, I mentioned that sugar holds about 61 different names and can easily be overlooked on the package labeling.

Perhaps you are trying to gain weight, especially in the thigh area (eek!). Or, you are okay with acne breakouts in your adult life (double eek!). In that case, load up on the sugary beverages because you will lose energy, gain weight, cause facial blemishes, and crave *more sugar*! That's right, folks. Sugar is similar to suppressant-like drugs, only it is not an illegal substance, unfortunately. It will trick your body into gaining weight by altering your metabolism. Sugar in the form of fructose, for example, does not appropriately stimulate insulin. As a result, consuming sugar will do absolutely nothing for your hunger-feeling hormones, called "ghrelin," and satiety feeling-hormones, called "leptin." Nonetheless, you will crave more sugary foods and develop a resistance to insulin all together. So, black coffee or tea is a way better option for an energy beverage than soda pop or energy drinks.

Oh, and don't forget about the mood triggers we discussed before. Sugar is likely to cause changes in your heart rate and metabolism. As a result, you will experience those up-and-down mood swing effects happening shortly after consuming high-sugar foods and beverages. I had this happen to me after indulging in a few pieces of chocolate fudge. Yay for the holiday season, right? Moods can be predicted and help you plan for expectation management if you are paying attention to your diet. For instance, a distant family member just had back surgery, and I was concerned about who

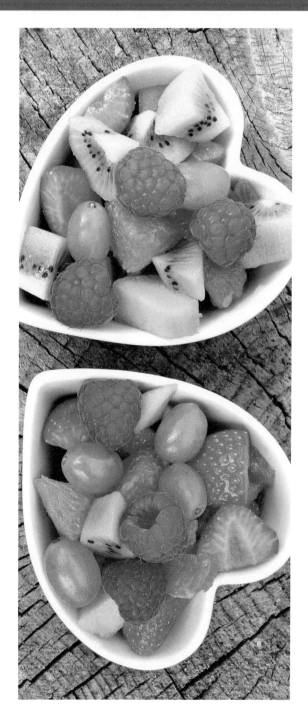

was going to take care of her while she was healing. A mixture of this stress, eating poorly, and skipping on gym is likely the cause of acne breakouts on may face, a common cold, and a urinary tract infection (UTI) to boot. And guys, this can happen to you too. This is basic human anatomy!

Okay, I can go on and on about how sugar can alter our body's overall shape and cause long-term health problems, but I think you got it at this point. Here is the good news for those with a "sweet tooth." Fruit has natural sugars that not only taste amazing but that also provide beneficial vitamins and nutrients that are essential for our bodies to function properly. Fruit can provide ample energy without unnecessary calories, provide adequate dietary fiber, and keep your digestive system regulated, as well as provide potassium in order to keep your blood pressure regulated. Vitamin C is commonly found in citrus fruits and known for boosting our immune system; healing wounds; creating healthy skin, teeth, and gums; and maintaining the lymphatic system. Refined sugars, on the other hand, are actually proven to weaken your immune system, which in turn causes you to become susceptible to the common cold. So, to parents who are reading this, pay attention to candy and sugary goodies that may be given out during school—bacteria and germs are festering there and our children's immune systems need to be up for the challenge. Stick with fruit for sweet treats like strawberries, blueberries, raspberries, apples, pears, pomegranates, grapes, and bananas, for example.

There are so many health benefits to eating raw fruits in terms of your overall heart health and digestive system. Antioxidant fruits, such as apricots, apples, bananas, cantaloupe, berries, grapefruits, and oranges are beneficial for heart health as they are rich in flavonoids, carotenoids, fiber, potassium, and magnesium. Fruits also provide vitamins like vitamin A, vitamin B6, vitamin C, vitamin E, vitamin K, and folate, all of which aid in regulating cholesterol levels and preventing diseases like stroke, atherosclerosis, and heart attacks. Specifically, expectant mothers may want to increase their fruit consumption as a rich source of folic acid. Folate is known to reduce the risk of neural tube defects, anencephaly, and spina bifida occurring during fetal development. I remember eating an entire fresh pineapple (face deep and definitely embarrassing) when I was pregnant with my daughter. It's amazing what your body naturally craves!

By now you are starting to realize that moods and foods are the foundation of your overall health. Eating raw vegetables and fruits literally cause a happier well-being—good food, good mood! So, when you need to keep going strong during a long work day, pack yourself a fruit-filled lunch with nuts and seeds for snacking. A light lunch with fruit, nuts, and seeds in the afternoon keeps your energy level up and naturally satisfies hunger.

I often get asked how eating a diet with so much fruit doesn't cause an imbalance in my blood sugar. With type 2 diabetes on everyone's radar across the globe, I can understand the concerns. Of course, a balanced diet is important, but in terms of fruits providing nutritional value for diabetics, your doctor may suggest eating fruits that have a low glycemic index to control your blood sugar level, such as apples, avocados, bananas, etc. Whatever works best for you in conjunction with your doctor's guidance is best, but generally speaking, raw and dry fruits are the best options for satisfying your appetite or sweet tooth. Keep in mind that the worst option for fruit you could possibility make are those fruits that were processed for packaging, such as canned or sweetened fruit cups. Anything processed, packaged, and prepared will have some sort of preservative in it to prolong the shelf life, as well as added sugars, which will never promote long-term health benefits.

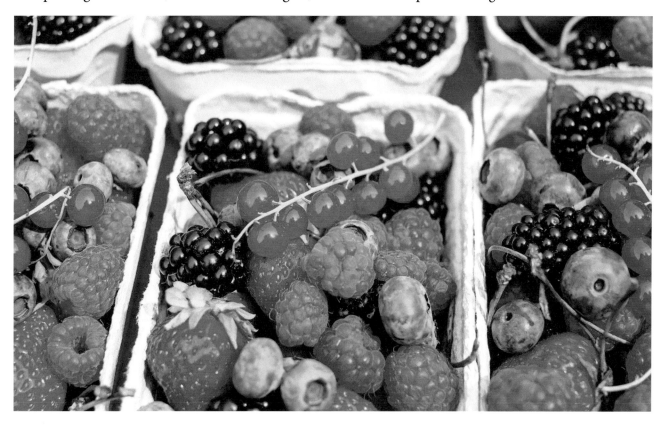

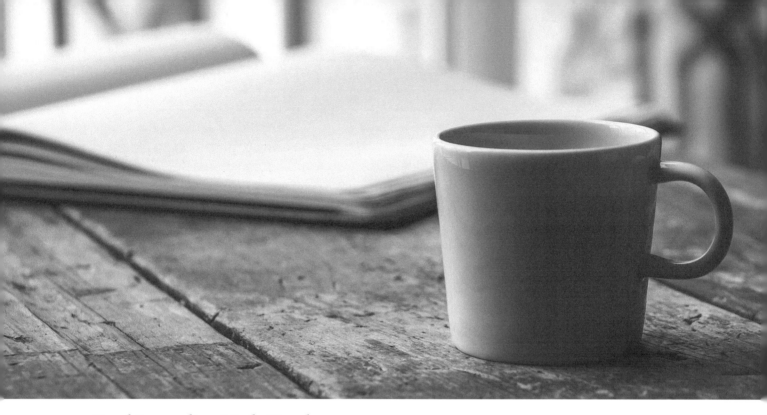

Food Journaling Made Simple

Growing up in New Jersey, I swore I was always going to be a vegetarian at age seventeen because I literally lived on pizza and bagels. Although I did eat some remnants of fruits and vegetables in my diet, dinnertime was more like an act of kindness. I grew up with a single parent who worked full-time while raising three kids, which is nothing short of admirable. And we never went hungry. However, I remember that chicken breasts were dry, beef roasts were overcooked and tough, and vegetables were usually the canned type. Everything was seasoned with salt and pepper—period. And if this doesn't sound like a common northeastern household, I will admit I looked forward to meatloaf and mashed potato nights because of the option to drown my food in processed, jarred, and very salty gravy. I thought I could live on bread and cheese and function just fine as a teenager, to be honest. Sure, there was the occasional prepackaged and seasoned beef tenderloin and imitation crab meat cocktail prepared once a year on New Year's Eve growing up in my house. The point is, as child I never developed an appreciation for the taste of meat, poultry, fish, or seafood, and so I claimed to be a vegetarian early in my adolescence. Now that I think about, this was not a bad situation since animal products are not the healthiest option anyway. However, I also grew up with extended family members who endured in the sport of deer hunting and always shared the venison with us—again, overcooked, very tough to swallow, and now with the wild gamey taste to displease my underdeveloped palate. I suppose it did not help that I worked at a local deli and bagel shop and had easy access to processed meats, processed cheese, bagels, and all the cream cheese you could really ever stomach. Ah yes, a classic favorite was an everything bagel with an inch of cream cheese on it. Don't forget the classic iced tea beverage (contains about 46 grams of sugar) to wash it down. It is perhaps still my favorite bagel option, but do I really need to eat 800-1000 calories before 8:00am in the morning? Not to mention, the starchy, grain-rich carbohydrates will sit in my stomach like a brick for about two to three hours, and I'll crave another bagel before my body can completely digest the first one. Bagels taste amazing—I get it. But I also know that I will feel sluggish after indulging in too many carbohydrates that take a long time to digest. This is the perfect example of why journaling your food could make a significant difference and really help you understand how food makes you feel. In this case, after eating a bagel I already know a few effects to watch out for—lethargy and uncomfortably full. Journaling can be as easy as keeping a food log on how you feel after consuming a food item with a few known facts already hardwired in your brain:

- I don't like feeling lethargic, weak, and unmotivated to complete tasks.

- I don't like feeling uncomfortable in my own skin or clothes.

- I don't like my mind and body feeling dull and lacking energy.

- I want to feel light, sharp, and motivated to complete tasks.

- I want to feel comfortable in my own body and feel confident wearing my clothes.

- I want my mind to be clear, focused, and full of energy.

Food choices can be tricky if you fall for that comfort food we all grew up with. Old habits are the hardest to change, especially if certain foods are a huge part of your culture and traditional upbringing. This is where I especially encourage you to keep a food journal. It will not take long to realize that certain foods like white breads, pastas, and sugar-based carbohydrates will have an effect on your body and mood. They are simple carbohydrates—that is, carbohydrates that are high on the glycemic index. The classic example of this is eating a candy bar to satisfy a craving. Be honest with yourself. How long did that satisfaction last after you ate the candy bar? Simple carbohydrates may digest quicker than complex carbohydrates, but they also have the potential to increase insulin and blood glucoses. I call this the "fast and crash" energy source. And we already discussed the dirty truth on sugar, or what I call the legal drug, in the previous section.

When journaling your food intake, really pay attention to the added sugars in your meals. Sauces and condiments are likely to have added sugars you normally wouldn't think about, like ketchup, for instance. Next time you see a bottle of ketchup, read the label and see what ingredients are listed. I bet you will find sugar as the second ingredient. In no time at all, you will find that common sugar-based foods, like cookies, pastries, ice cream, and all those treats you crave, will start to correlate with a sluggish and unmotivated body. It's the start of the vicious cycle that can lead to feelings of stress, irritability, and depression. Okay, maybe that is an extreme example for eating one simple Christmas cookie during the holidays, but become absolutely mindful of how many cookies you indulge in and how often. Remember, sugar is an addictive drug; it can never satisfy your body's need for nutritional calories, and you are setting your body up for fat gains. Here's how it works:

- A rise in glucose leads to a rise in insulin, which will likely result in fat gain.

- Your body slows down the process of burning fat for fuel and continues to add glucose to fat and muscle cells.

- Since insulin moves glucose from the blood to fat and muscle cells, it can leave you feeling unenergetic and tired.

A whole-grain bagel, on the other hand, is considered to be a complex carbohydrate (low on the glycemic index) because of its ability to be absorbed and released into the bloodstream a bit more slowly; hence the digestion process is slower as well (Mercola 2010). Raw vegetables, quinoa, oatmeal, whole-grain pasta, sweet potatoes, and beans are better sources of carbohydrates for this reason. Physically eating slower will augment the digestion time for complex carbohydrates. So essentially, eating a diet rich in fiber, protein, and healthier fats a lot *slower* will assist you in feeling complete satiation.

Food journaling can be a bit time consuming and a tedious process. Several apps are available to expedite this process if you have a smart phone. And if you have a fitness tracker, or a product that collects your personal data, calories burned, heart rate, sleep patterns, and so on, even better. For those not interested in food journaling who just want a nutritional diet baseline of choices to choose from, you are in luck—keep reading. Of course, with variety and moderation, I will provide a basic list of foods to choose from over others. But first, it is important to understand what you are looking for in the grocery store and the reasons it matters. So let's start with the fat choices.

Fat Choices

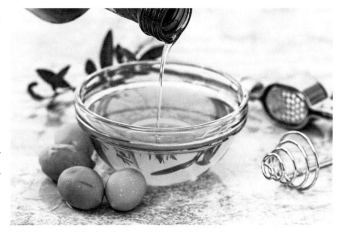

Here's the skinny on fat. When including fat in your diet, you have to pay attention to calories. That is, there are 9 calories per gram of fat. These calories do not fill you up very easily. To include fats in your diet, avoid any processed or refined fat sources when cooking, baking, or frying. Pretty simple, right? Well, it would be simple if there were not so many different types of fat sources to choose from. I personally like the taste, soluble consistency, and nutritional value that comes from extra virgin olive oils, but it is not necessarily the best choice for cooking certain foods. At the very minimum, I try to avoid processed vegetable, canola, and corn oils at all costs based on how I will feel after eating them. My gut will feel bloated and cramped, and I will most likely have a headache shortly after eating restaurant-style fried chicken tenders and French fries. Fried chicken and potatoes alone would be great, but the processed vegetable oil it was fried in will cause all sorts of discomfort, namely bubble guts and a head ache. Also, most people believe that a vegetable salad is a great option for a meal. I would totally agree with this, but I would also argue that the salad dressing used on your salad could cause some health setbacks. For example, even though you chose to use olive oil and vinegar on your salad over the creamy ranch dressing, understand that oil is still a fat source and should be used sparingly!

In a perfect world, I would love to live on fresh avocados, raspberries, almonds, broccoli, spinach, and salmon based on the nutritional value and health benefits of these foods. Seriously, these are all super foods that are packed with everything you need for a healthy, balanced diet. Unfortunately, our culture and social environment influences us to think we need to cook with some sort of fat source for almost every meal. For example, do you use cellophane materials or Teflon brand cookware? Do you commonly use nonstick oil spray products? Well, I would consider researching the toxicity and health risks associated with nonstick pans. Then, ensure you read the label on any type of sprayed-on oil source and avoid consuming additional chemicals with your meals. It is a lot to think about just to keep your fried egg from sticking to your pan. Instead, invest in a black iron cooking pot, as I have found it is the healthiest way to go. No one should ever have to worry about potentially consuming metal particles or chemical compounds in their food. I use a table spoon of extra virgin unrefined olive oil in a black iron Dutch oven and have no issues with any food sticking to my pan. By doing so, I avoid metal-like materials chipping off in my food, and I can adequately measure the amount of fat I am cooking with. Remember, even though I believe extra virgin unrefined olive oil is best choice, I am still aware that it is a fat source.

Fat options can be overwhelming and confusing when determining what is best for which type of cooking method. Why not have an organized list to refer to? Below is a list of commonly used fat sources with their best associated uses and best nutritional facts. The values are based on a 2000-calorie diet, so your values may change depending on your calorie needs. These common fat sources are found in most households for cooking, baking, and general uses. Pay attention to the "means of use" as most processed foods will have a fat source listed in the ingredients on labels. There are certain fat sources I would avoid altogether based on overall health outcomes.

Note: This is my personally complied list of common fat sources used in a household for cooking, baking, and other means of consumption. It is not a complete list of fat sources available. Nutrition values are indicated and may vary.

Best Fat Sources	Best Means of Use	Nutrition Highlight
Olive oil	Stovetop cooking, baking, frying, sautéing, salad dressing	Virgin, extra virgin, pure Vitamin E and vitamin K Anti-inflammatory 14 grams of fat/serving
Coconut oil	Stovetop cooking, taking off facial make-up	Virgin (organic), unrefined, pressed Increase energy Early sense of satiety 14 grams of fat/serving
Hemp seed oil (Manitoba harvest)	Add drops to enhance nutrient content, salad dressing	Anti-inflammatory High omega-3 and omega-6 13 grams of fat/serving
Peanut oil	Deep frying based on high temperature tolerance (frying a turkey), roux base, homemade tortillas	Increase energy Polyphenol antioxidant High omega-6 13 1/2 grams of fat/serving
Sesame oil	Stir-fry, sautéing, salads	4 1/2 grams of fat/serving
Flaxseed oil	Tablespoon added to salad dressing or smoothie	High fiber 4.3 grams of fat/serving
Ghee (unsalted clarified butter)	Cooking, baking, sautéing, spreading	Grass-fed livestock Vitamins A, D, E, and K High omega-3 and omega-6 22.7 grams of fat/serving
Butter (salted/unsalted)	Cooking, baking, sautéing	Grass-fed livestock 14 grams of fat/serving

Best Fat Sources	Best Means of Use	Nutrition Highlight
Hazelnuts	Snacking, salad topper	High energy source, vitamins E and K 17 grams of fat per 1 oz.
Almonds	Snacking, salad topper	Rich in vitamins E, K, and magnesium 28.35 grams of fat per 1 oz. serving
Walnuts	Snacking, salad topper	18.49 grams of fat per 1 oz. serving 3.89 grams of carbohydrates/ serving 4.32 grams of protein/ serving
Pumpkin seeds	Snacking, salad topper	Mostly polyunsaturated fat 9 grams of fat per 1 oz. serving
Avocados	Best eaten fresh/whole	Vitamin C High energy source 29.47 grams of fat/serving 17.1 grams of carbohydrates/ serving 4.02 grams of protein/serving
Sunflower oil/seeds	Snacking, salad topper	13.6 grams of fat/serving

Other Fat Sources to Avoid	Means of Typical Use	Nutrition Highlight
Vegetable/canola oil	Baking	Rapeseed organic Rapeseed conventional 13.6 grams of fat/serving
Soybean	Stovetop cooking	Genetically modified 13.6 grams of fat/serving
Coconut oil	Stovetop cooking, baking	Hydrogenated/refined 14 grams of fat/serving
Butter (salted/unsalted)	Cooking, baking, sautéing	Grain-fed 11.52 grams of fat/serving
Margarine	Spreading, baking	Hydrogenated Ingredients vary 3.77 grams of fat/serving
Shortening (regular or butter flavored)	Butter replacement	Vitamin E 12 grams of fat/serving
Corn	Stovetop cooking	13.6 grams of fat/serving
Palm/palm kernel	Skin and hair care	Vitamins E and A 13.6 grams of fat/serving
Lard	Pates, sausages, pastry fillings	High monounsaturated fat Side effects: headache, drowsiness, irritability, dizziness, vomiting, lethargy, diarrhea, and bulging of fontanels in infants 12.8 grams of fat/serving

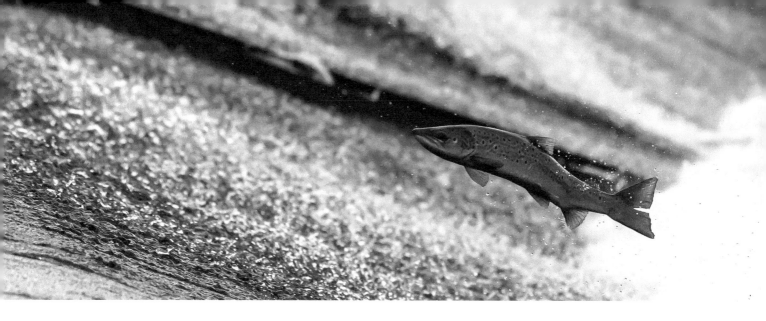

Wild versus Farm-Raised Salmon (and Other Fish)

Ah, yes, those perfect days on a sports fisherman boat and reeling in the freshest catch of the day have forever changed my thinking on eating fish, or any type of seafood for that matter. I wasn't always so grateful for harvesting anything from the sea, as I am the one most likely to puke or get a fish hook in my eye. Seriously, if the ocean water has a slight ripple in its movement, my head is hurled overboard and nausea takes over the rest of the day at sea. After netting my first king salmon in Sitka, Alaska, I got over the motion sickness pretty quickly. Nonetheless, reeling in something fresh is rewarding, and it tastes better than store-bought fish; plus, I appreciated it more since I knew the process that took place before serving it to my family. I will try not to get all scientific with you in this segment of the chapter, but salmon are so important to our diet and life cycle. From eating wild instead of farm-raised salmon to comprehending spatial aspects of where our fish came from, I will definitely encourage you to rethink fish in your diet.

It is uncommon to visit your local grocery store and stop and think about the process that took place prior to your physically buying fish, meats, or anything really. You may actually lose your appetite in the middle of the aisle if you ever stopped to think about the processing that chicken or types of red meat went through before being put on display to buy. In fact, if you took the time to watch *Vegucated*, I am sure that you would find that the vegan diet is not that extreme and seems completely reasonable. Nonetheless, stay with me as go through some key facts about salmon, and if it doesn't meet your palate's needs for one reason or another, try to increase fish consumption in your diet at the very least. Here's why.

Process—it is so important to comprehend where your food comes from. What body of water did your fish live in? How it was processed, packaged, and shipped to your area? And yes, discussing salmon is necessary because this species, in particular, is a critical component to your health and our environment. I'll explain.

Scientific data and research of wild and farm-raised salmon species has shown that there is appropriate risk communication that balances the health benefits of consuming salmon (e.g., physical health and cultural subsistence) with the health risks of consuming salmon that may contain metals and persistent organic pollutions (POPs). For the most part, research is pretty constant on finding that the health benefits from consumption of salmon and fish oil outweigh the health risks based on the correlation of salmon nutrients—which richly consist of omega-3 fatty acids and proteins—and the reduction of cardiac heart disease (Lall 2010).

Health risks associated with salmon consumption varied based on the harvest region and whether or not the salmon was farm-raised or wild caught. For example, according to researchers, there were higher concentrations of polychlorinated biphenyls (PCBs), polychlorinated dibenzo dioxins (PCDD), polychlorinated dibenzo furans (PCDF), and organohalogen pesticides in European wild-caught salmon species. Also, it is common for researchers to discuss the effects of fishmeal in accordance to case studies. Farm-raised salmon are more likely to be contaminated with high levels of dioxins in the European regions than other Western regions based on the fishmeal content used to feed salmon in fisheries (Lall 2010). Keep in mind that fishmeal reveals both health benefits and risks. Significant research indicates that most fishmeal and fish oils are induced with animal byproducts, enhanced protein supplements, genetically modified ingredients, antioxidants, ground-up marine animals, and sometimes growth hormones. However, fishmeal ingredients are regulated by the US Food and Drug Administration (FDA) to ensure there is no, or minimal, impact on human health. Interestingly, most research discusses higher levels of methyl-mercury bio-accumulates found in wild-caught salmon in contrast to farm-raised salmon (Fairgrieve and Rust 2003). It is quite a lot of biology to realistically think about during a grocery run, but at the very least, understand there is a clear distinction between farm-raised seafood and wild-caught seafood.

Overall, it is no secret that salmon is proven to be a high source of protein and omega-3 fatty acids that promote cardiovascular health. Those who consume salmon should always read labels when making a purchase at the local supermarket. Research consistently shows that wild-caught salmon from Pacific regions contains fewer persistent organic pollutants (POPs) than salmon harvested in northern Atlantic regions. Also, wild-caught salmon are more likely to be exposed to contaminants from commercial fishing, cleaning, shipping, and processing activities. Farm-raised salmon will be fed fishmeal for a three-year period before being harvested, may contain dioxins, and are more likely to be exposed to water-borne diseases from fisheries (Lara, et al. 2006). And finally, there are several different salmon species that all have a unique taste to them, as well as texture and color differences. With all this said, Pacific Coast wild-caught salmon that I personally caught and processed is fundamentally the best choice overall options.

Below is a table of common salmon species we generally see on our plates and their nutritional value. Next time you are in a restaurant ordering salmon, impress your dinner date and ask, "What type of salmon are you serving tonight?"

Table 1. USDA Nutrition Information for 100 (g) of Cooked Farmed and Wild Salmon							
	Calories	Protein (g)	Fat (g)	Saturated Fat (g)	Sodium (mg)	Cholesterol (mg)	Omega-3 (g)
Farmed							
Atlantic	206	22.1	12.3	2.5	61	63	2.1
Coho	178	24.3	8.2	1.9	52	63	1.2
Wild							
Chinook (King)	231	25.7	13.3	3.2	60	85	1.7
Sockeye (Red)	216	27.3	10.9	1.9	66	87	1.2
Coho (Silver)	139	23.4	4.3	1	58	55	1
Pink (Humpback)	149	25.5	4.4	0.7	86	67	1.3
chum (Keta)	154	25.8	4.8	1	64	95	0.8

(Tom and Olin 2010)

Salmon are also major transporters of invaluable nutrients for not only human consumption needs all over the world but also for substantial coastal, lake, and riparian ecosystems as well. Through anadromous processes, or the spawning process, high accumulations of marine-derived (MD) nutrients, consisting primarily of nitrogen, phosphorous, and carbon, are transported by salmon activity. Although these nutrients are essential for human and animal life, salmon are found to provide a nitrogen source that stimulates algae growth as well (Moore et al. 2007). Furthermore, the soil near coastal, lake, and riparian zones is found to be thicker and richly saturated with MD nutrients where salmon are likely to spawn. It is found that these zones attract a prosperous living habitat for plants, insects, fish (including salmon species), and scavenger animals, such as the coastal brown bears that may carry salmon away. Research analysis explains that the coastal, lake, and riparian ecosystems not only benefit from the deposits of salmon eggs and carcass decay, they also benefit from the physical activity of salmon nest-digging while spawning. Through monitoring salmon activity during periods of spawning, studies have proven that salmon are major transporters of MD-nutrients (Moore, et al. 2007). So, for my gardening enthusiasts, get yourself a bucket of salmon guts or a fish carcass and burry that in your gardening soil. I bet you will have a successful gardening seasoning!

Spatial aspects and anthropogenic catastrophic events within areas of spawning salmon are proven factors that may alter salmon populations, as well as the transport of MD-nutrient content. It is common for biologists to connect a salmon population decrease to spatial aspects. For example, there are potential risk factors that impede on chinook salmon populations in the Puget Sound, Washington, where there were geographical impacts from landslides, earthquake activity, hatchery release, and facilities leaking and spilling toxins. These anthropogenic effects are found to assist MD-nutrients' transportation as well as transport persistent organic pollutants (POPs) and toxic chemicals, such as pesticides, dioxins, polychlorinated biphenyls (PCBs), and polycyclic aromatic hydrocarbons (PAHs) (Naiman et al. 2002). In relation to anthropogenic catastrophic events, some research has determined that these toxins are found in the groundwater near Pacific Ocean waters and are responsible for a decrease in the salmon population, as well as subtle effects such as liver disease, reproductive damages, and immune system disruptions (Good et al. 2008).

For Alaskan communities, harvesting salmon is so important that the Alaskan native culture is defined by it. Subsistence fishing and commercial fisheries are also significant for communities as they provide a major food source and a variety of employment opportunities that support local economies. Salmon are a vital part of the food chain within most Alaskan territories throughout every stage of the salmon life cycle. Cold, clear streams, lagoons, lakes, major rivers, estuaries, and the open ocean are all occupied by salmon species at some point in their life cycle. All of these habitats must remain stable to sustain a healthy fish population.

Salmon is by far a favorite in our household. The health benefits of wild-caught salmon outweigh those of farm-raised, and it is considered a super food due to its nutritional value. Eating a diet high in omega-3 fatty acids and vitamin D is known to improve bone health and brain function, promote heart disease, improve eyesight and skin, and boost the immune system. For eating, I prefer sockeye (red) salmon and chinook (king) salmon based on taste and texture. Coho (silver) salmon is also a common favorite but, in my opinion, is best prepared in the smoker. See Chapter 7 for smoking preparation and cooking techniques.

Cooking Methods

Cooking salmon should not be an intimidating concept. There are so many flavors to season it with, but cooking techniques for any fish depend on the thickness of the filet. First, let's assume you have gotten past the catching, purchasing, or acquiring the filet of choice and are ready for the preparation process. I will break down the basics here for those who need the preparation steps. Otherwise, if you are beyond that skill level, then just skip over to the recipes to start learning how to include more fish and vegetables in your diet.

Steps to Fish Preparation

1. Defrost your filet, if necessary, in the refrigerator, ideally overnight. This will ensure that bacteria does not collect on your filet as it sits on your counter or in a water bath.

2. Once you have the filet defrosted, use a deboning tool, if you have one, to remove all the bones. I previously used my husband's needle-nose pliers for years until I broke down and bought the five-dollar tool. What a difference it makes when pulling out salmon pin bones.

3. Okay, pay attention here if you don't like the fishy flavor, especially if plan on cooking it with the skin left on. Regardless of whether you process your own fish or buy from the store, rinse off the filet with cold water and then pat dry with a paper towel. This is also the perfect opportunity to trim up the filet and use that deboning tool again if necessary.

4. Coat the filet with olive or coconut oil—your choice—and season as desired. I like to use a combination of sea salt, black pepper, cayenne pepper, and garlic powder. Lemon pepper seasoning and premixed fish seasonings work as well, but be cautious of the sodium content in premixed seasonings. Also, once you get to the bottom of a premixed seasoning container, the majority of the contents will be mostly salt. Over salting your filet will likely leave you disappointed and deter you from ever adding fish in your diet.

Once you have your filets all prepared, you can decide on the cooking method. Here are a few of cooking methods for salmon, halibut, and rockfish that I use often.

Salmon: Season as detailed above and blacken for about two minutes on each side. I like to let the skin get crispy enough to eat since it holds a good portion of fat nutrients, which are great for your health and cell membranes. Another delicious choice for salmon is to season your filets with fresh lemon, fresh garlic, and sea salt. Then bake your filets on an aluminum-lined tray or baking dish at 375 degrees F for about twenty minutes or until done.

Salmon Poke: This is perhaps my favorite way to prepare salmon, although you will need to freeze fresh-caught salmon for at least seven days to ensure that all the bacteria and potential parasites are killed. I have prepared sushi before with freshly caught salmon and wolf eels and I survived, but it is best to practice food safety and not risk the potential contamination of food-borne illnesses. So, for all raw recipes when using fresh fish, ensure you allow freezing time before preparing any dish. See Chapter 6 for the full salmon poke recipe.

Halibut: Season as detailed above and blacken for about two minutes on each side. I would avoid frying or blackening halibut thicker than one inch, as this type of white fish is lean and will dry out quickly. Look for a moist and flaky consistency when you cut with the side of your fork. You should clearly see the layers of the meat separate easily. Season with fresh lemon, fresh garlic, and sea salt and bake at four hundred degrees for about twenty minutes or until done.

Halibut Olympia: Make sure your filet preparation steps 1-4 are complete, but filets are a bit thicker than 1 inch. Large halibut filets can be as thick as 2-3 inches. For halibut Olympia it is important to cut the fresh filets into a 3-inch by 4-inch cube, then slice the cube into ½-inch layers - think lasagna-layering techniques but no more than three layers. There are three main recipe trends for the Olympia filling that include either using mayonnaises, sour cream or cream cheese as the filling base. I only use homemade kefir cream cheese and add fresh green onions with a mixture of fresh minced garlic, Worcestershire sauce, lemon pepper seasoning and Tabasco sauce. Bake at 400 degrees F for 25 minutes.

Rockfish, cod, other white fish: Filets are normally pretty thin, so I like to sauté this type of fish meat in a black iron skillet with olive oil, coconut oil, or a grass-fed butter source. Seasoning is your choice, but any salt source will be soaked up in the meat fairly quickly. Use salt sparingly. These are a perfect choice for fish tacos! Baking instructions are similar to salmon as detailed above, but filets are usually thinner and will need less time.

Game (Organic) Meat or Nothing at All

I first started out by stating that the best guideline to follow to kick-start a healthy lifestyle is to adopt a diet of plant-based foods in their rawest form possible. Then, I went on to talk about wild-caught fish as the better choice over farm-raised, and now, I am about to discuss meat choices even though we all have a general idea of the adverse health effects of animal products. Why am I not totally sold on a plant-based diet? Well, the fact is, I know that a plant-based diet is the healthiest choice, but just like most Americans, I am addicted to eating animal products— meats, poultry, fish, milk, cheese, butter, eggs, the list goes on. Whether we argue that eating animal products is socioeconomically acceptable or find government-driven incentives to eat them, most Americans find it difficult to cut animals completely out of their diets. That being said, I am a realist and willing to admit that I love the taste of red meat, and I am also aware of its direct linkage to heart disease. I still crave steak. I salivate over the smell of bacon and eggs in the morning. I continue to pour milk in my children's cereal when I am in a pinch for time. I use butter occasionally when sautéing foods, and I enjoy all seafood; fresh poke' and sashimi are high up on my favorites list. I am not proud to admit these cravings, but animal foods have been a part of my culture since I can remember. I am sure it is the same for most of you reading this right now. So, I will be realistic in my attempt to support a plant-based diet and encourage you to minimize red meat or any animal product consumption. Here's how.

Mindfulness is the key factor that will support healthier food choices. For instance, I am more mindful of how often I consume animal products and more motivated to maintain a plant-based diet because I continue to educate myself on what it is exactly I am eating. I ensure that educating myself on healthier food options is a priority because, well, I want to avoid cancer, heart disease, high blood pressure, high cholesterol, and any other chronic illness that is preventable. I want to be healthy enough to see my children go to college. I want to live a healthier life, so when my children have children of their own, I will be active and able to be a huge part of their lives. And so, I encourage every meat-eater to think about their meat sources differently after reading this section. If you are not into eating any animal products at all, congratulations on setting the right example. But keep reading anyway because there is a valid, educational argument that you will appreciate.

Wild game is the freshest, healthiest meat source there is available in our world today. I know this is a bold statement, but just stop and think about the process a restaurant-served hamburger went through to be all dazzled up with lettuce, tomatoes, cheese, and that favorite condiment you like to add. It is likely made of ground-up feedlot cattle that are fed mostly genetically modified organism (GMO) corn and soybeans along with a heavy dose of antibiotics and probably started its journey on a meat farm factory. But I digress on government food-producing incentives and specifics from the meat-processing industry.

Think about this instead. A subsistence lifestyle brings you all things organic and whole with minimal processing of wild animals to that desired burger on your plate. Sure, it takes a certain character to feel absolutely comfortable killing a live animal (or fish for that matter) just to be gutted out in the middle of the woods and packed out by way of your back. I get it. This is not typical food shopping for everyone. Mindfulness of the processing that took place of your meat source is really the only point you need to remember here. In my opinion, if I cannot kill my own fish and game, then I really do not even want to eat it. But life happens, and we find ourselves shopping for meat, poultry, or fish at the grocery store anyway. It is imperative to carefully read the labels and figure out how long the food product took to get to that commercial grocery store. If certain preservatives have been added to meat products, it is best to not eat them at all. There are some brands that do their best to avoid adding nitrates, for example, to their processed meat products. And if you are new to the latest research on nitrates, then do your homework. Processed meats are full of sodium nitrites to preserve meat products. Sodium nitrite is also a chemical found in some explosives, which is alarming, but I digress again. Anyway, nitrites are also linked to immobilizing brain development in children. The point is, I would rather know that I am eating a deer that lived in the wild eating organic grass its entire life rather than risk eating a carcinogenic piece of bacon. As you may have predicted, I avoid feeding my children any processed deli meats, sausage, or packaged meat products altogether. Yes, I am completely okay with depriving my children of ever eating a hot dog.

Every food item we put in our mouths has been through some sort of processing. Food-borne illnesses and chronic diseases are more likely to affect our lives if we trust the meat-processing industry wholeheartedly to feed us. It is no secret that processed meat is commonly associated with adverse health effects such as increased carcinogenic risk factors that are directly linked to colorectal cancers, heart disease, and other chronic diseases (Harvard T.H. Chan 2019). At the very least, be mindful and read the labels on hot dogs, ham, bacon, sausage, and most deli meats that have been treated in a way to preserve or flavor it. Processing that generally occurs in these types of meats includes salting, curing, fermenting, and smoking. Keep in mind that red meats include beef, pork, lamb, and goat. Read your labels carefully and avoid excessive additives and preservatives at the very least if you absolutely need to satisfy your meat craving.

Regardless, animal products are not really necessary to support and maintain a healthy diet. We can always find the necessary nutrients from vegetables, fruits, legumes, nuts, and seeds, but we commonly choose to eat what our society and environment deem acceptable. I accept wild fish and game in my diet, and I am mindful of how often I consume it. I try to avoid red meats and poultry entirely, and I primarily eat fish and vegetables. This was not always my diet, but cancer and heart attacks are common adverse health concerns in my family; therefore, I need to pay attention to my genetics, as well as my diet, closely.

At the very least, all meat variations and poultry should be considered side dishes, and the main focus of your meal should be the vegetables you consume. If you have consistent traces of high blood pressure or anxiety, then you will find a plant-based diet most helpful in controlling those health concerns. As always, consult your doctor for diet guidelines if, in fact, you have high blood pressure, anxiety, or heart-related concerns. Since animal products are not the healthiest food sources and you may not be into hunting, fishing, or a subsistence way of life, then consider cutting animal products or, at the very least, red meat out of your diet completely.

CHAPTER 4:

ACTIVE LIFESTYLE THAT WORKS FOR YOU

Clearly, not everyone is an absolute fitness freak. In fact, only a small percentage of Americans consider physical fitness to be a priority in their daily routine. Sure, it may be easier for some to commit to an exercise regimen than others, but raising your heart rate for ten to twenty minutes a day will increase your confidence and focus and help maintain a less stressful lifestyle. If you cannot commit to ten to twenty minutes every day, make the effort to do something requiring intense functional movement or focus on a single activity. Everyone can find a moment to walk up a stairway a few times or lift a few boxes from a storage closet. No excuses! Your personal active life may entail a yoga session, walking in the park, riding a bicycle to work, painting your latest masterpiece, landscaping your lawn, or working on a house project. Even a moment of coloring with your children will provide natural endorphins if you focus long enough on it. Focusing on one task will allow you to become more mindful and more confident so that you can handle any obstacle or mood trigger that comes your way. And if you detest any activity that makes you sweat, meditation practice will do the trick. Whatever your physical activity is for the day, make sure you make it your top priority. An active lifestyle means actively engaging your body *and mind* in order to get those natural endorphins flowing. Staying active is different for everyone but so critical to include in your day in order to maintain a healthy balance.

For my gym-goers, do not get hung up on body image when you think about living an active lifestyle. It is important to understand that looking healthy is based on body image, and bodybuilders are not always the healthiest people. The fact is that, no matter how many back squats I do or miles I run, I will always have my genetics to thank for that inherited love handle layer on my hips. Although I enjoy circuit training and endurance running, my body is naturally shaped like a gymnast and not a runner. (Too bad I am far from ever becoming a gymnast!) The point is that I have grown to love my curves and accept the imperfections as they define me. In the same way, every intricate part about you is beautiful and unique. And if you cannot see that within yourself right now, you will after you start feeding yourself better food choices. Remember, good food equals a good mood! Consider the caterpillar who has to wait to become a beautiful butterfly: she has to eat and is not afraid of the metamorphosis process. Understanding yourself and accepting the beauty you have is life-saving. So before you spend any more time obsessing over body image, know that you have the ability to control things like food choices and your environment, and these two major factors can change your body and mind fairly easily.

Okay, so you have decided to get moving and need to decide which fitness program is right for you. There are hundreds of health and fitness programs to choose from today. Social media sources do not make it any easier since our commercialized culture is designed to make you a believer in everything sexy. You ladies know damn well you just bought those Lululemon leggings and suddenly got inspired to tell Shaun T. how to shake it. I am guilty of online browsing just to get motivated to get active and escape a lazy funk. I call this my retail therapy! Whatever attire gets you motivated to move, social media sources can overwhelm your social media feeds the moment you "like" whatever trendy athletic wear catches your eye. Do not get sucked into the nuances that the fitness industry promotes. Remember, you are in control of food choices and your environment. That also means you are in control of your finances as well, so be cognitive of what you spend on your active lifestyle goals.

The health and fitness industry has expanded so much that most people find themselves overwhelmed with fitness training programs and nutrition guidance. Likewise, a poll taken from Facebook and Twitter users determined a list of the top ten most-searched fitness programs. CrossFit was ranked number one, with 65 percent of men searching the Internet for a workout of the day (WOD). Yoga, Zumba, Insanity, P90X, Couch to 5K, SoulCycle, Squat Challenge, kettlebell workouts, and plank exercises were the other top ten programs. The most popular fitness program in 2016 was Les Mills, followed by the Tracy Anderson Method, Jillian Micheals Body Revolution, the Body Beast, Tone It Up, LiveFit, the Daily Burn, the Bar Method, and SurfSET Fitness. The online Bodybuilding.com brand alone lists over fifty different workout programs for you to choose from to meet your health and fitness goals (Find a Workout Plan 2019). Oh, and let's not forget about the ever-growing popular training programs solicited to you from online entrepreneurs who absolutely believe that Beachbody, for example, is the only one to follow. I actually think Beachbody has a great approach for marketing its effective wellness brand because it uses everyday people making health a priority in their lives. All these fitness programs I have mentioned are very effective, and the fact that you have already chosen one of them or even recognize any of them is awesome news in itself. Continue doing what works for you and try to recruit your loved ones to stay active as well, no matter what definition you have for living an active lifestyle. Maintaining an active mind and body every day in some capacity relieves stress and enables you to make better food choices and, above all, healthier life decisions.

I could not include a motivational section on fitness without mentioning the providential and auspicious creation of miracle pills and weight-loss shakes. Those who feel they need to drink a pre-workout shake or swallow a genetically modified supplement in order to get motivated to move are at risk for far more adverse health outcomes than those that do not use anything to get motivated. More than half of the adult population of Americans has taken dietary supplements to stay healthy, lose weight, gain an edge in sports or in the bedroom and avoided using prescription drugs to do so (Gahche et al. 2011). Supplements and performance products are overwhelmingly popular within the fitness industry. There are some pre-workout products out there that consist of natural, organic ingredients, but it is common to find sugar as additive as well for taste value. Read labels on everything and be mindful of the potential added metals in protein shakes and pre-workout products. What most Americans do not realize is that there is lack of oversight on the production of dietary and performance supplements. That is, the FDA has not exhausted its authority granted by the (industry-friendly) 1994 Dietary Supplement Health and Education Act (DSHEA) to ensure products are safe and do not have adverse health effects. Despite our lack of education on supplements, Americans spent $26.7 billion on dietary supplements in one year, according to the *Nutrition Business Journal* (Fox 2010). If you need energy and motivation before heading to the gym, try eating an avocado, an apple, or some nuts and drink plenty of water. Most supplements will strongly advise drinking plenty of water with the product anyway because of their potential to cause dehydration. Eating the right energy foods will be easier on your digestive system and less strenuous on your liver, heart and kidney function as well. Again, what are we accepting as food? Supplementing a meal with a protein shake may provide the results you are looking for, in terms of body image, but do you really know exactly what you are consuming?

Here is a list of a few common energy foods I normally eat before an intense 20 to 30-minute high-intensity workout:

- One avocado, one plum tomato chopped, one tablespoon of olive oil, and sunflower seeds

- One half cup of any nut or seed combinations (cashews, almonds, walnuts, pecans, macadamia nuts, etc.)

- Any fruit choices (apples, pears, oranges, cantaloupe, melon, various berries)

- One cooked sweet potato or one-half cup of seasonal squash

- One half cup of cooked oatmeal, walnuts, raisins, dates (optional: add one tablespoon of raw honey if you need it to be sweeter)

- One cup of black coffee (when I am desperate for energy!)

So now what? We are surrounded by so many health and fitness influences, and everyone seems to have the most effective health and fitness methodology or philosophy—for the right price, of course. The truth is that you do not need an expensive training program to improve your health. Learning to be more interconnected with your body's response to food and exercise can avoid an anxiety attack the next time there is a 5K fun run in your town. Sure, personal trainers help optimize your time and effort to reach your personal health and fitness goals, but you have to be sure to include all those factors in your life that make you balanced. A nutritional diet, mental stimulators, personal interests, and of course having fun are all very important to include in your fitness program or activity of choice.

Whatever activity trend you are following, most people find that community fitness is a major motivating factor. From an empowerment perspective, humans are hardwired to naturally gravitate toward community environments that make us more advanced—healthier, stronger, or whatever definition of *advanced* works for you. High-intensity fitness programs, similar to CrossFit, Insanity, P90X, or my personal favorite, Street Parking by Julian and Miranda Alcaraz, are among the community fitness programs that help hold you accountable for achieving your fitness goals. Why does Street Parking work best for me? It is a workout program that not only is tailored to personal physical abilities but also can be done anywhere while using minimal equipment. I am a mom of two young children and currently living in a very remote area. My "me time" is between 5:00 a.m. and 6:00 a.m. when nothing happens in my household. The Street Parking program offers daily online exercise coaching, nutrition meal plans, community support, and affordability. Let's face it—we all share a common goal to look good naked! I do not have time or resources steadily available to me as other people may have living in a more urban community. With that said, below are a few realistic tips to supporting a more active lifestyle.

Choosing a Fitness Program: Ask yourself what is most important in your life. Perhaps you have a family history of heart disease—the number-one cause of death in Americans by the way (CDC 2017)—and you want to live a healthier lifestyle for your children. Perhaps you have been battling weight loss your entire life and depression has taken over. If changing your lifestyle is important, then finding a fitness program that fits your needs should be your highest priority. Community fitness programs are a great way to help find your preferred fitness program by simply talking to people who care about your overall health and will support your fitness goals.

Nutrition: Clean eating is eating only things that are, in fact, real food! Preservatives, hormone enhancers, and chemical additives found in processed foods are sure to stay in your gut longer, have minimal (if any) nutritional value, and most likely slow you down. Refined sugars and sodium nitrates are usually the main culprits and are found in most processed foods. Try to eat fresh, raw produce more often in your diet.

Personal Awareness: Read food labels and become aware of what ingredients you are consuming and how you feel after you have eaten them. Gaining awareness of how your body feels after exercising and eating certain foods provides you with a basic foundation to feeling better about yourself. Once you start understanding how your body reacts to certain foods, you will know what to avoid and what to consume to improve overall health and performance. Above all, be realistic with your goals! An easy way to keep yourself on track is using the commonly used **SMART** approach:

Specific: A specific goal has a much greater chance of being accomplished than a general goal.

Measurable: Establish concrete criteria for measuring progress toward the attainment of each goal you set. Ask yourself if it is really weight loss you seek or perhaps you are researching to feel mentally and physically better than before.

Attainable: When you identify goals that are most important to you, you begin to figure out ways you can make them come true.

Realistic: To be realistic, a goal must represent an objective toward which you are both willing and able to work.

Timely: A goal should be grounded within a time frame. No timeline means no urgency to make healthy changes in your life. Focus on meeting a deadline, and you will surely push yourself to achieve that goal.

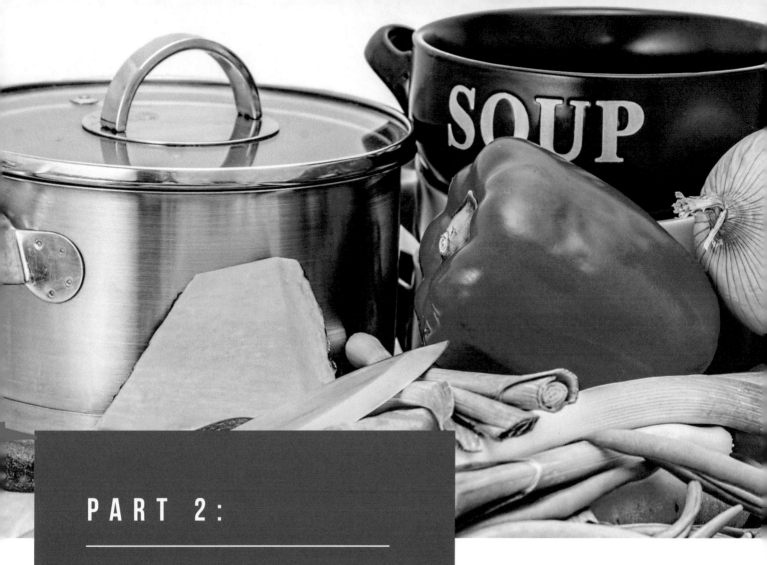

PART 2:

COOKING RECIPES FOR REAL WHOLE FOODS

CHAPTER 5:

SELF-HARVESTING ALWAYS WINS

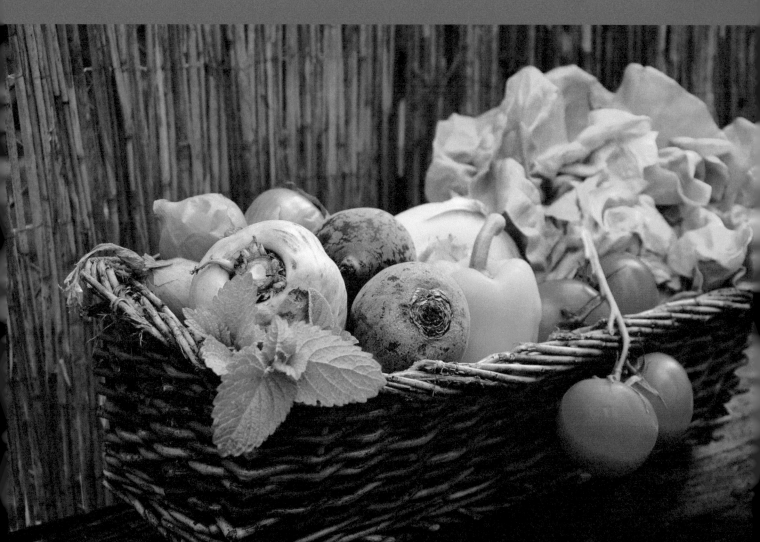

If you enjoy a lifestyle that enables you to effectively garden, gather, hunt, or fish, then you will reap the health benefits from self-harvesting for almost no cost at all. Not everyone enjoys digging in the dirt to grow food or can fathom taking the life of an animal, but the health benefits of doing so outweigh grocery shopping every time. Research reveals that 95 percent of farm animals, such as chickens, pigs, cattle, and turkeys, in the United States are raised in farm-factory conditions (ASPCA 2019). The factory conditions and processing methods are enough to make anyone think twice about that delicious burger from their favorite restaurant, as I mentioned already. With that said, it is important to respect those who hunt and fish in terms of necessary subsistence and cultural meaning.

I actually put myself through a thirty-day self-harvest challenge, and it was nothing short of gratifying. Why endure such a challenge? It was perfect for my environment and daily schedule and incorporated things I love to do in Sitka, Alaska (i.e., fishing, hunting, gardening, and berry picking). This thirty-day challenge was intended to examine how I feel on a particular diet, experience the impact of clean eating for myself, and provide a real example for journaling food choices to include in this book. More importantly, I wanted to provide an example for you in hopes of influencing your decision regarding a plant-based diet. The challenge was not aimed at weight loss, but rather forced me to think about how I felt after thirty days of absolutely clean eating. Learning to garden efficiently and understand caloric intake were major highlights to this challenge. Unexpectedly, I also came to appreciate the true essence of respecting fish and game subsistence practices.

So here is what was on my menu that was actually self-harvested:

- **Fish and game:** halibut, salmon, venison, and rockfish

- **Garden vegetables:** kale, French lettuce, butter lettuce, broccoli, potatoes, rhubarb, green onion, and garlic

- **Herbs:** cilantro, dill, mint, Thai basil, and sweet basil

- **Fruit:** salmon berries, blueberries, raspberries, and huckleberries

The only foods bought from the grocery store in support of the thirty-day self-harvest challenge were coffee beans and seasonal fruit. I used olive oil or coconut oil and dry seasonings for cooking and preparing meals.

I was interested in studying how my body would respond to a purely organic diet provided from the environment in which I live. I intended to eat only local foods, physically feel the difference in my mood and energy levels, and journal the changes once all preservatives and food-processing additives were no longer in my body. I have always found myself to be more energetic and gain mental clarity while keeping up with a whole-foods diet, although this self-harvest challenge brought new variables into the equation. I did not have access to eggs, chickens, pigs, or a variety of nuts; therefore, I was only left with what I could personally grow, catch, kill, or gather.

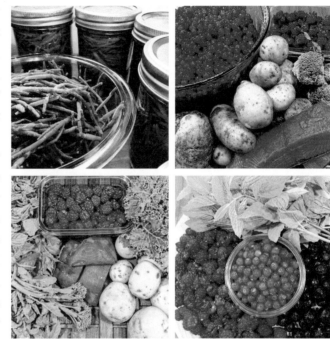

What has always been interesting to me is that everyone has a different body type and everyone responds to certain diets differently. In the past twenty years, regardless of exercise regimen, my weight has always been consistent with the exception of two pregnancies. What has changed significantly, though, is the shape of my body, both internally and externally. I can easily feel the difference in my body if I drink alcohol or eat processed foods almost immediately. Besides feeling a bit bloated in my jeans or sluggish the next day, depression is expected as well after indulging in a night of drinking and overeating processed foods. So why do we repeat these food-binging behaviors? It's not enough to say it is human nature to enjoy tasty food and overeat. Unfortunately, our brains are hardwired to remember things that taste good. Plus, our culture encourages us to be the social beasts that we are, and most people love to eat and drink.

You have heard the saying "You are what you eat," and I cannot explain just that in a more simpler way. I have repeatedly mentioned to health enthusiasts that how we feel and perform is primarily based on what we accept as food choices. Staying active is just as important, but good eating habits give us the fuel to be energetic in our daily lives.

When I used a self-harvested weekly meal plan for thirty days, I put my personal theories of clean eating to the test. For my own sanity, I made black coffee and used store-bought fruit (only apples, bananas, and pears) and a variety of dry seasonings as exceptions to the self-harvested menu. The results of the challenge that I recorded are as follows.

Week 1: July 25–30

I am feeling more energized than I've ever felt as I reach day seven of the thirty-day challenge. The only setback is underestimating how important it is to increase calorie intake if you are working

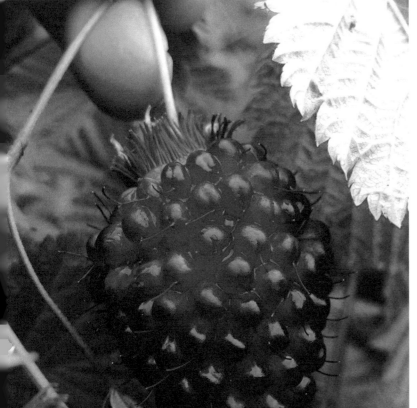

out. Instead of draining myself completely, I decided to maintain the self-harvested food plan and hold off on intense and heavy workouts until the challenge is over.

My cravings for salty foods are crazy and, unfortunately, my carbs are only garden veggies and berries. I am absolutely grateful for adding black coffee and store-bought fruits to the meal plan at this point. Another variable to the challenge is competing with garden slugs on my lettuce, deer stomping through my garden beds, as well as rainy, cold weather in Sitka, Alaska. This has not only caused slow growth in my garden, but I also had to harvest the lettuce much earlier than expected. My body has definitely responded in terms of headaches—most likely from sugar withdrawals—and a heightened sense of smell. I ate raw mint leaves simply because they smelled good and were easy to grab while walking my dog one morning.

Week 2: July 31–August 6

This week the challenge took a turn for the worse. The slugs absolutely decimated both butter lettuce and French lettuce crops, and the deer literally ate four of nine broccoli plants to the ground by day eleven. The Brussel sprouts and spinach are growing slower than expected, and so I still haven't been able to harvest them at all at this point.

Although I stopped heavy lifting in my daily workout routine to reserve my energy, the kale, broccoli, sea asparagus, and added fruit alone have not been enough calories to sustain me. I am eating apples, as well as the apple core, and mint leaves for snack meals. I can easily eat an eight-ounce smoked salmon for a snack without thinking twice about eating the skin as well. I absolutely need to berry pick daily to sustain the amounts of calories I need to function clearly and feel energized. I am constantly thinking about food and, literally, salivating over my toddler's apple scraps. At this point, I am concerned my body is using muscular tissue and stored fat. I am even more concerned for my ability to function safely for my children since I am normally a very active mom. There is a clear lesson learned here that plant-based calories are digested much faster, and I underestimated how much I actually need to sustain energy. It is evident that eating more plant-based foods in your diet will potentially broaden the gap between health disparities and inequalities as it costs more to eat fresh produce than other processed food sources.

Week 3: August 7–13

I thought day seventeen of the challenge may be the end based on the lack of garden vegetables and berries, but the weather pulled through. A full week of sunshine was enough to keep a steady harvest of kale, broccoli, lettuce, potatoes, and the substantial amounts of raspberries and huckleberries daily. Just in time too, as the salmon berry season just ended.

The best source of energy I have available that is both satisfying and fulfilling is smoked salmon bellies. The fat on the salmon is a perfect source of calories needed in a meal choice. A common mistake that people make, in terms of caloric intake, is that 1 gram of fat = 9 calories, whereas carbohydrates and protein calories each give you 4 calories per 1 gram. Cutting fats completely out of your diet will be challenging if you want to sustain high energy to function every day. The other important variable to keep in mind is complex versus simple carbohydrates in your diet. All my garden vegetables are enough carbohydrates to sustain the energy I need, although my metabolism is burning through the harvested meals much quicker; I have to eat more carbohydrates to stay energized than I did before. Again, this is the perfect example of how food disparities and inequalities are increasing among populations. That is, maintaining a healthy diet can be costly and almost impossible in some parts the world. Thus, processed foods may fit the grocery bill but also increase the risk of chronic diseases, such as obesity.

Week 4: August 14–23

It is day twenty-five, and I am feeling really good about being able to add a substantial amount of broccoli, kale, potatoes, and raspberries to my meals. Even my family is supported with a plentiful harvest to consume healthy calories as well. Then, I discovered that the deer depleted (and trampled on) the Brussel sprouts, broccoli, and some kale plants. At this point of the challenge, I am thankful for the frozen sea asparagus, canned salmon, and pickled sea asparagus I prepared prior to the challenge. If I had to solely rely on my garden for carbs, I would have had to end the challenge within eight days. I have gained an even greater appreciation for fishing, hunting, and gardening during this experience, all while feeling disappointed that one deer trampling on my garden can change the fate of the entire self-harvest challenge.

These last few days have tested my discipline and will, whereas I seriously started to imagine subsistence living in far worse conditions. I keep reminding myself that my culture has shaped my eating behaviors, where food has always been available in some form of a grocery store, restaurant, or other means of buying food. Food dependence is something we often take for granted. I am truly grateful to gain the full experience of self-harvested meals and undoubtedly understand the health benefits of clean eating because of the way I feel—energized and focused.

Lessons Learned: I am more conscientious of the amount of food needed to sustain energy. I never really counted calories before or even thought about food portion size until now. I literally needed an entire cup of berries to feel satisfied and gain a usable, healthy source of energy. I am a busy mom of two; I do not have time to measure and weigh food portions, but it was easier to consume the perfect amount of food for meals when I used fresh fruit as snacks.

I have much respect for farmers and gardeners since harvesting food is time consuming and calls for intense preparation. Canning salmon, rhubarb, and sea asparagus prior to the challenge was critical to make it successful. Sure, you can be creative with how you cook meals with seasoning, but I literally ate three-gallon-size bags of sea asparagus, about thirty-five cups of various berries, eighteen jars of canned foods, and everything that was edible from the raised garden beds during this challenge.

This challenge was not about weight loss; however, my internal body has changed significantly. Yes, my waist is leaner and has more toned muscle definition as a result from clean eating, but my complexion is the clearest and smoothest it has ever been. The greatest internal change is my mental clarity. I am much more driven and can focus easily on things that once felt overwhelming at times. I am no longer craving sugar, processed foods, or alcohol. I thought I would never pass up a cold stout or a glass of pinot noir! As mentioned before, sugary foods actually increase dopamine levels and leave you craving more calories. Eliminating sugar, processed foods, and alcohol eventually helped my brain forget about taste and enabled me to crave anything that supported energy. As a result, I actually started to crave smoked salmon and raspberries during the challenge.

Growing and harvesting my own food has been nothing short of an amazing and gratifying experience. I hope to inspire others to seriously think about the benefits of eating real, whole foods and appreciate the greater value of fishing, hunting, and gardening as an encompassing, total body balance. Eating fresh produce rather than processed food is saving lives as plant-based foods and clean eating are the best health trends that are making headway.

CHAPTER 6:

HEALTHIER MEAL OPTIONS

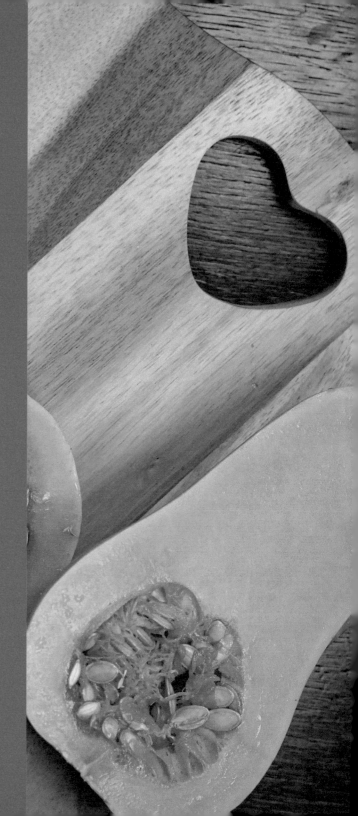

Diet trends can be just as overwhelming as the fitness industry I mentioned in Chapter 4. It is common to read about trending diet plans that guarantee weight loss if, and only if, you use their products to augment the process. In other words, a business based on selling you *their* products. Do you plan on taking dietary supplements for the rest of your life? Of course not; it is just not sustainable to do that for a long term. Sure, there are other diet plans that are supported by science, such as the Mediterranean Diet, Paleo Diet, Vegan Diet, and of course, the Gluten-free Diet, namely. There are also several different Belief-based Diets that encompass religion and culture. Based on medical research, I would agree that there is a need to implement specific diets for one reason or another. For example, a doctor may prescribe a specific diet for weight control for a diabetic or a Gluten-Free Diet for a patient that has been diagnosed with celiac disease. All these diets have a place in our society when under the respective conditions. For most people who have not been diagnosed with a medical condition, it is best to just eat a plant-based diet – real whole-foods. Try to avoid extreme diet plans that claim rapid weight loss or consuming dietary supplements. Your body is not a vessel for experimenting; so why treat it as though you are in a lab? If you are eating whole-foods that are in its' rawest form, then you are sure to be able to maintain this type of healthier diet for life.

I have to admit—I do more food preparation than fancy cooking techniques or food presentation. I really do not care what the food looks like, to be honest. I care about how the food will affect me after it has been consumed. The taste is definitely up there on the importance scale, but I am mindful about cooking the nutrients away in the process and losing the authentic flavor of the food item itself. Let's use French fries as a classic example. Deep-frying white potato wedges in vegetable oil may be ideal for that crispy texture you aimed for, but the actual taste of the fries will be of that vegetable oil. Also, the deep-frying process will always increase your fat consumption.

Try this instead: For French fries, wash and cut sweet potatoes into wedges, toss in a bowl with a tablespoon of olive oil and seasoning of your choice (e.g., salt, pepper, and garlic powder), spread on a baking sheet lined with parchment paper, and bake at 400 degrees F for thirty minutes or until they are of the preferred texture. Again, more preparation time will be needed, but it is a healthier option. This method of preparing and cooking any vegetable is simple, easy, and a healthy way to ensure that most nutrients are preserved throughout the cooking process. I usually add onions and peppers to the baking sheet or deep glass dish for additional flavor.

Baking Sheet Directions for Vegetables: Wash and cut vegetables, toss in a bowl with a tablespoon of olive oil and seasoning of your choice (e.g., salt, pepper, and garlic powder), spread on a baking sheet lined with parchment paper, and bake at 400 degrees F for thirty minutes or until they are of the preferred texture.

Here's a list of common vegetables that can be cooked up using this baking sheet method with preparation modifications based on type of vegetable.

Sweet potatoes	Cubed, sliced, wedged (baked or roasted)
Yams	Cubed, sliced, wedged (baked or roasted)
Acorn squash	Cut in half, remove seeds, add olive oil/seasoning, turn over with skin up, bake as directed
Spaghetti Squash	Cut in half, remove seeds, add olive oil/seasoning, turn over with skin up, bake as directed
Seasonal winter squash	Cut in half, remove seeds, add olive oil/seasoning, turn over with skin up, bake as directed
Butternut squash	Cubed, use glass dish for roasting (will likely be soft)
Brussel sprouts	Remove first few leaves, prepare for baking sheet
All pepper types	Add to any baked/roasted vegetable for additional flavor
Kale	Rip apart into finger-length pieces and prepare for baking sheet
Zucchini	Cut into ½ inch strips and prepare for baking sheet

Dips, Salads, and Soup Variations

Too often, I find myself attending house parties with delicious sides and dips that I just cannot resist. You know that anything made with cheese is a crowd pleaser. Oh, and do not forget the mix of alcoholic beverages to really dull your senses on counting how many times you actually indulged in someone's fondue fountain. Guilty here on all counts. And you know what else? I am usually the culprit holding a bottle of wine jumping at the chance to fill your glass. I suck at self-control at social events. Food, alcohol, whatever—keep it coming until my husband literally has to take me home. I have gotten better on the alcohol consumption mainly because I always remember how much I do not enjoy hangovers. But tasty food never gets old, so I made it a priority to bring tasty, healthier food options to house parties. No, it is never a good idea to bring kale salad to a Thanksgiving potluck. That will surely cause you to be cut off the upcoming Christmas list. You can, however, bring a festive salsa or ceviche dish that will be the highlight of everyone's night. For some reason, we humans always enjoy chopped-up anything with salt on it. Why not make it chopped vegetables with salt and lime, for example?

Regardless of the house setting or ambiance, next time you find yourself invited over for a dinner party or gathering, bring something you know will be guilt free. Time should be spent socializing and visiting, not feeling a tremendous amount of after-party blues. Seriously, I can remember punishing myself after a night of heavy drinking and binge eating. After the hangover cleared, I would try to remember what I ate the night before just to get motivated to sweat it out in the gym. Next weekend, repeat. This is the fast way to destroy your liver, gain weight, and do who knows what else I was actually doing to myself both mentally and physically.

Self-control is a concept I am still trying to work on when it comes to food choices. Cutting down on alcohol (and other recreational drugs, if you partake) helps clear your mind to make better food choices. Here are some of my favorite recipes for foods I like to take to house parties and potluck-type gatherings to avoid the next-day food guilt vibes.

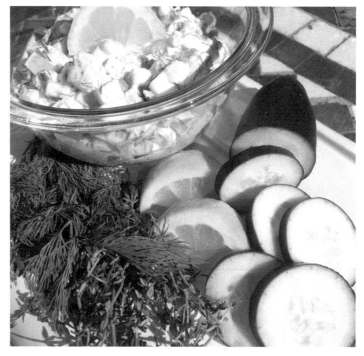

Cucumber Salad or Dip

Maintaining physical and mental balance is based on about 90% of what we eat, so I am going to provide you with a few comfort-food choices. Healthy comfort food is possible and is a must (at least for me) as there so many ways to eat tasty whole foods to settle our snack-head cravings. Comfort food is my happy place because - let's face it - we all eat and congregate in the kitchen as human beings. So, here is a simple, healthy side dish that will impress your guests and will certainly be a crowd pleaser.

Here is what you will need:

- 2 large cucumbers, diced

- 1 bushel of green onions, diced

- 2 tablespoons of fresh dill, diced

- ½ teaspoon fresh thyme, diced

- Juice of 1 lemon

- 1/2 cup of plain kefir (substitute with plain Greek yogurt if kefir is not available)

- Lemon Pepper seasoning to taste (salt, black pepper, lemon zest seasoning)

Directions: First, prepare the cucumbers, greens onions, fresh dill and thyme in a bowl that will allow you to gently mix with a spoon. Add lemon juice, kefir, then seasoning and mix well. The cucumber salad is ready to eat immediately, but dish becomes more flavorful and watery over time in the refrigerator.

Note: You can cut off the pits and skins of the cucumbers, but I try not to waste anything in my cooking techniques. If the cucumbers are washed well, why not gain the nutrients in the skin and pits too? Fresh ingredients make all the difference in this dish. Serve with your favorite tortilla chip or eat plain as a side salad.

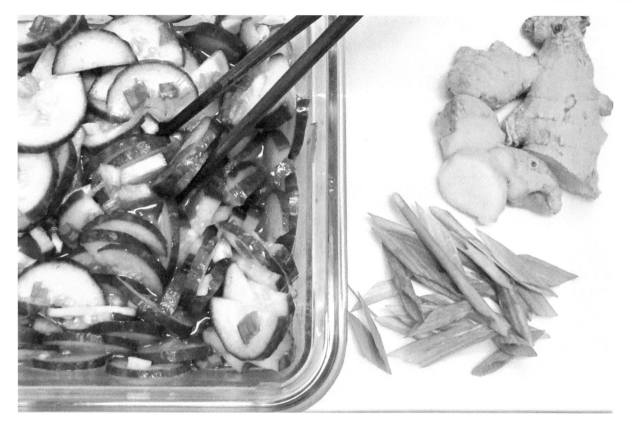

Cucumber Kimchi Recipe

This Korean-inspired cucumber side dish will be your favorite once you taste it. I absolutely love Korean bulgogi lettuce wraps and all the fixings that go with them, but finding a cabbage kimchi in rural Alaska was a challenge for me. Forget about preparing fresh spicy red Napa cabbage kimchi out here (preferred choice) due to the lack of fresh produce and time to ferment properly. It is best to leave that up to experts in Seoul. Plus, who doesn't love cucumbers?

I actually adapted to a more spicy-like palate some twenty years ago and have never looked back at those Northeastern salt and pepper taste buds. This recipe is full of flavor and gives you the ability to turn up the heat however you like. Once you prepare all the ingredients below, it is absolutely ready to eat. That is the beauty of this recipe. The flavor is spot on immediately and requires minimal *whole* ingredients. Real food that tastes really good—give it a go!

Here is what you will need:

- 2 English cucumbers, sliced into half circles

- 3–4 green onion stalks, diced

- 1/4 cup of finely diced fresh ginger

Note: Other cucumber types will give you more seeds and will water down fairly quickly. If you cannot find them, no worries. This dish does not last that long anyway.

Kimchi Sauce

- 2 tablespoons Sriracha pepper sauce to taste

- 2 tablespoons rice vinegar (or white vinegar)

- 2 tablespoons sesame oil

- 4 tablespoons raw honey

- 2 tablespoons of fish sauce

Note: Do not use apple cider vinegar unless you like tangy, zingy, and pucker-causing kimchi.

Directions: Prepare the cucumbers, greens onions and ginger separately and set aside. In a separate bowl whisk the kimchi sauce ingredients until you reach the desired level of spice. Once the sauce is prepared, pour over chipped the cucumber, green onion and ginger. The cucumber kimchi is ready to eat immediately, but dish becomes more flavorful over time in the refrigerator.

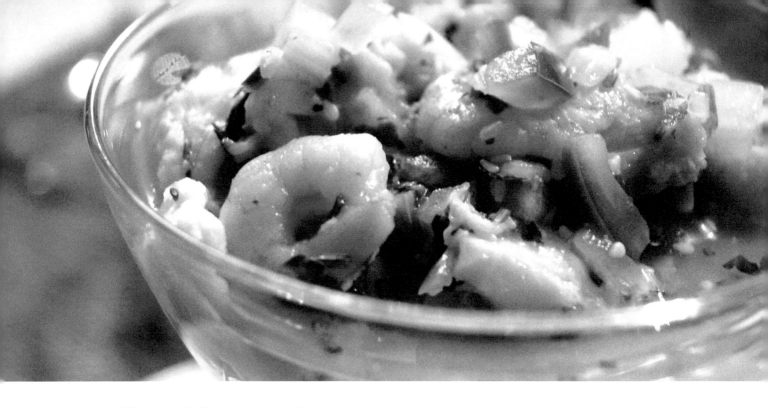

Halibut and Shrimp Ceviche

This recipe is perfect for large house parties but involves some preparation. The first point to make here is that any white fish will work pretty well with ceviche dishes. Keep in mind how the fish was processed and remember to use fish that was frozen for a week or so to kill any bacteria or parasites. If you want to use fresh fish and skip the freezing process, there are food-borne illness risks associated with eating raw fish, but since ceviche is cooked (so to speak) by the citrus in the lime juice, you will likely be okay. It's your choice.

Here is what you will need:

- 2 pounds of Halibut or other raw white fish, diced

- 1 cup of peeled raw shrimp, diced

- 3 jalapenos, diced

- 3–4 Roma tomatoes, diced

- ½ **bushel of** fresh cilantro, diced

- Juice from 2–3 limes

- Salt to taste

Directions: Combine all ingredients in a large bowl and refrigerate for about two hours to ensure the lime juice cooks the raw ingredients. Serve with your choice of tortilla chips.

What is the Deal with Kale?

How do you make something delish with kale? Well, first let's explain some variations of kale types because I feel like kale has a bad reputation. It is common to hear that people buy certain types of it and use it for the wrong reasons, which is easy to do because various types of kale that are geographically unique. Well, here is a simple breakdown on common types of kale you will most likely see at the grocery store or at your local market. Kale is absolutely a super food that you must try to include in your diet and here is why.

Kale contains vitamins A, C, and K as well as minerals and disease-fighting antioxidants that will literally make you feel good from the inside out. Kale has the antioxidants, like carotenoids and flavonoids, that have been found to protect against certain types of cancer. Also, kale is a low-calorie, high-fiber, high-iron, and zero-fat kind of food source. It is a leafy green food that cleans out your intestines and helps process some toxic foods you may have lingering in your gut (Szalay 2015).

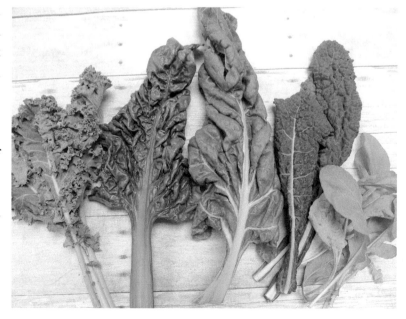

What type of kale to eat and when.

1. Curly kale or Redbor kale: This type of kale feels like sports turf and is probably the most common kale sold in bunches at your local grocery store. Because of its tight, ruffled leaf-like structure, it holds up great in the oven when baked. I use this type to make kale chips for my kids pretty often. **Directions:** On 1 bushel of chopped kale, massage 1 tablespoon of olive oil throughout. Then lay out the kale on a cookie sheet, add sea salt and garlic powder, and bake for about 20 minutes (or until crispy) at 350 degrees F.

2. Red Russian kale: Great for adding to a spinach or field green-type salad. The leaves are smooth and flat but difficult for your stomach to digest because this type of kale is so robust. There is a hint of a spice in this kale, as well.

3. Lacinato kale: This is also known as dinosaur kale and is my favorite type to use in preparing a kale salad. Also, it has a robust texture and is full of nutrients. I will provide a great recipe that really makes this type of kale work perfectly regardless. It has a slightly sweeter and nuttier taste than the types mentioned above. Following is my favorite kale recipe that works well for lunch, a dinner side dish, or a house party favorite.

Kale Salad Recipe

When it comes to making kale taste good, it is all in the dressing. There are so many variations of kale salads. Trying to wrap my head around a go-to recipe was a long and trying process, but I think I figured out my favorite by using Royal Gala apples, sweet baby peppers, and my homemade dressing.

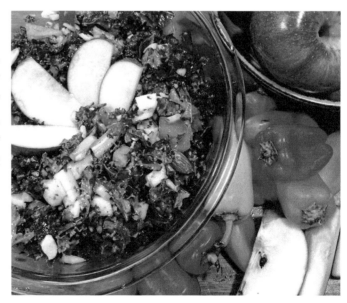

Here is what you need to chop up and toss together.

- 1 bushel of Lacinato kale

- 2–3 Royal Gala apples, peeled and cubed

- 8–10 sweet baby peppers (red, orange, and yellow), chopped

- 1/2 cup red onion, diced

- 1 cup of walnuts or other nuts, halved

- 1/2 cup of cherry tomatoes, halved

- 1 can of chick peas (garbanzo beans), drained

Homemade Lemon and Honey Dressing

Here is what you will need for the dressing:

- Juice of 1 fresh squeezed lemon

- 2 tablespoons of raw organic honey

- 1/4 cup of olive oil

- salt and black pepper to taste

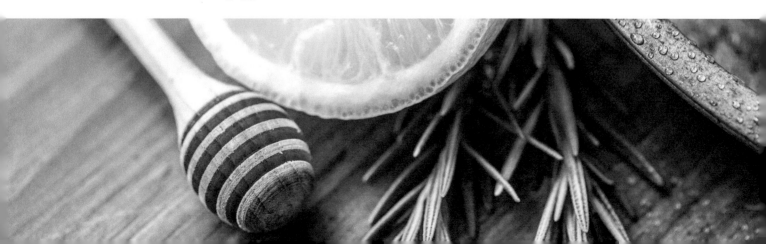

Directions: Prepare the vegetables above separately and set aside. In a separate bowl, prepare the Lemon and Honey Dressing and ensure all honey is completely mixed well by using a whisk. Once the dressing is prepared, pour over the vegetables, apples, and desired choice of nuts. The kale salad is ready to eat immediately, but dish becomes more flavorful over time in the refrigerator. I recommend doubling the batch of dressing to give the kale salad a bolder taste. You can use this salad dressing recipe as a chicken marinade or vegetable dipping sauce too.

Costa Rica Salad

I remember my husband coming back from a month-long trip studying in Costa Rica and raving about the cabbage salad he ate there. I tried to reinvent his experience and bring an authentic dish to our table, but the name just stuck—Costa Rica Salad. It is really not a salad in the sense of eating with a fork from a bowl or plate; rather, it is more like a salsa that we literally cannot stop eating. I have been bringing this recipe to house parties for over a decade ever since, so I will share this easy recipe so that your guests will love it too. I promise!

Here is what you will need:

- 1 head Asian Napa cabbage, diced
- 1/2 cup red onion, diced
- 3–4 jalapenos, diced
- 1 green bell pepper, diced
- 3–4 Roma tomatoes, diced
- ½ **bushel of** fresh cilantro, minced
- juice of 2–3 fresh limes
- 2 tablespoons of white vinegar
- salt to taste

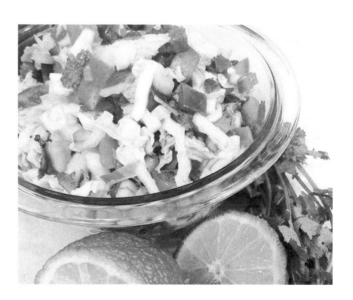

Directions: Mix all ingredients together in a large bowl and let sit for about 30 minutes to allow the lime and salt to do their magic. It's literally that easy and ridiculously delicious. We normally eat it like a salsa with tortilla chips or add to our breakfast eggs.

Squash Soup (Acorn, Butternut, Japanese Squash)

Don't overthink soup variations, and never forget the power of the slow cooker. Time is everything, and I do not like to spend more than ten minutes preparing vegetables for dinner. Using a slow cooker, or an Instant Pot if you have one, cuts your cooking time in half, but you will always have some sort of preparation to do regardless of what you make for dinner. Here is a quick power meal that is vegan friendly and has a unique balance of flavor.

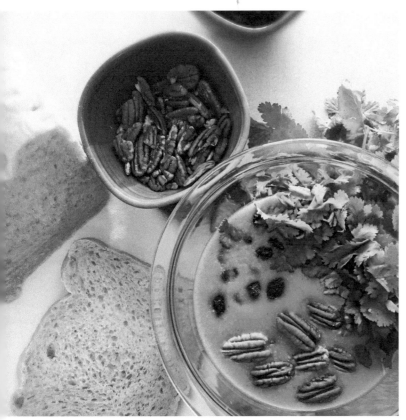

Here is what you will need:

– 1 whole acorn squash or butternut squash, peeled and cubed

– 1 can of organic coconut milk

– 2 cups organic vegetable stock

– 4 Gala apples, peeled and chopped

– 2 tablespoons turmeric

– 1 tablespoon cinnamon

– salt to taste

Note: If you don't have vegetable stock on hand, you can use 2 bouillon cubes and 2 cups of water. The apples and squash of choice will provide some water to the crockpot as well.

Directions: Put all ingredients in the slow cooker and cook on low for about 8 hours. The ingredients will be chunky; to create a smooth texture, transfer some of the contents to a blender and pulse until smooth. Pour back into the slow cooker and repeat until all chunks are smooth and blended well. Garnish with fresh cilantro, pecans, apples, and raisins.

Vegetable Pho

Pho is so quick and tasty! And the best part is that it is easy to skip the time needed to chop up fresh veggies if you buy a bag of frozen stir-fry vegetables. I know—I am always reminding you that fresh is better. Honestly, time spent preparing your meals should not deter you from consuming adequate vegetable portions. I get it, and it is perfectly fine to skip the fresh produce to make a healthier meal happen in a timely manner. Remember, the nutrients in frozen vegetables are the same as in fresh vegetables.

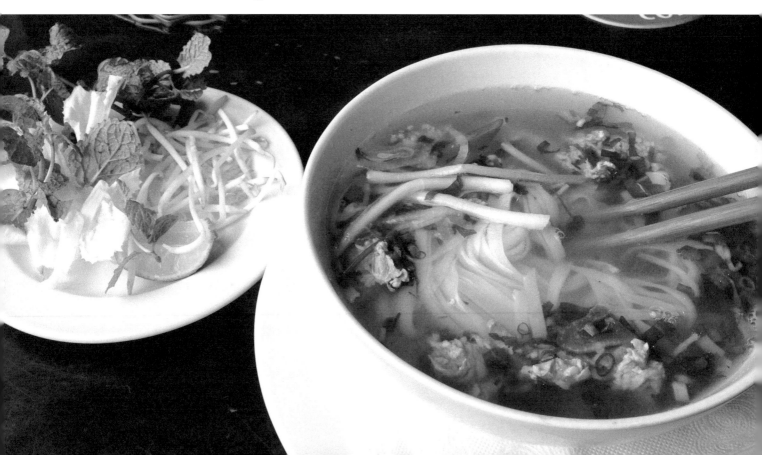

Here is a quick recipe for vegetable pho, although I am sure someone who makes authentic Vietnamese pho may not agree. Look folks—sometimes we just need good food on the go. I absolutely love authentic pho with all the right traditional veggies (and meats and seafood), but I threw this recipe together in ten minutes.

Here is what you will need:

- 2 tablespoons of sesame oil
- 2-3 cups of your choice of fresh or frozen vegetables, chopped
- 1 teaspoon of oregano
- 1 teaspoon of thyme
- ½ teaspoon of basil
- ½ teaspoon of rosemary
- salt to taste
- 1 bushel of fresh green onion, minced
- 1 tablespoon of minced fresh ginger
- ½ a head of cabbage

Note: I use half a bag of frozen stir-fry veggies with broccoli, sugar snap peas, orange/yellow carrots, mushrooms, red bell pepper, and water chestnuts.

Directions:

1. In the sesame oil, sauté the vegetables in sesame oil until tender in a deep, black iron pot (Dutch oven). I use the black iron Lodge brand pot.

2. Add oregano, thyme, basil, rosemary, and salt.

3. Add green onion, ginger, and cabbage.

4. Once the vegetables are cooked to your liking, set aside to make the pho soup liquid separately.

Pho Soup Liquid

- 4 cups of stock (vegetable, or beef stock works great, but use whatever equivalent stock you have on hand)

- 3 tablespoons of fish sauce

- 3 tablespoons of Sriracha

- Juice of 2–3 limes

Directions:

1. Mix all ingredients together in a medium bowl.

2. Pour the pho soup liquid into the iron pot with the veggies and let simmer for a few minutes.

3. Serve with quinoa or spiral-cut zucchini if you have time to spare instead of traditional pho noodles or rice. Quinoa is great source of dietary fiber to help with digestion. Quinoa is also the better choice over any type of rice. It takes 15 minutes to cook up a cup of quinoa. Enjoy!

Spicy Shrimp Pho

Perhaps my favorite pho recipe morphed into what it is today by a simple ingredient—fresh shrimp from Southeast Alaska. Using sesame oil is key for a real pho broth taste. Use the sesame oil to sauté garlic cloves and add your favorite chili paste as you see needed for flavor.

Here is what you need to add to your pho soup pot:

- 1 teaspoon of coriander seeds

- 1/4 teaspoon of ground cloves

- 1/2 teaspoon of black peppercorns

- 2 tablespoons of fresh ginger, minced

- 1/2 tablespoon of chili garlic paste

- 8 cups of organic vegetable broth

- 1 teaspoon of lemon zest

- 2 tablespoons of fish sauce

- Juice of 1 lime

- 2 tablespoons of hoisin sauce

- 1 teaspoon of cinnamon

- 2 pounds of raw shrimp, peeled

- 1 bunch of kale or bok choy, chopped

- 1 cup of shiitake mushrooms, sliced

- 1–2 zucchinis for spiraling into noodles (optional). Rice noodles work well too.

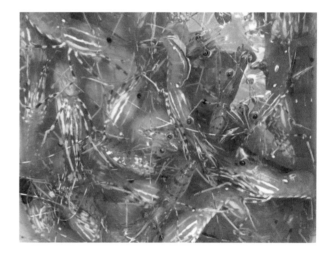

Directions: Mix all ingredients together in a soup pot and cook on your stovetop on medium for about 20-30 minutes to ensure all ingredients are mixed well and flavor had some time to set in. Most traditional pho recipes add a rice noodle, or bánh phở, but as always, I would influence using a vegetable spiral tool to make noodle-like pieces out of the zucchini. Garnish the pho with fresh jalapenos, cilantro, lime wedges, bean sprouts, and Thai basil. Add Sriracha or hoisin sauce to taste as desired.

Salmon Poke

Salmon poke is simple to prepare and provides a great source of protein, omega-3 fatty acids, and a great source of vitamin D. Sockeye (red) salmon is the best choice for sushi-type meals based on the texture of the meat itself. Salmon, in general, is a sturdy meat that holds up with most cooking methods, including grilling, baking, broiling and blackening in an iron pan. But for the purpose of preparing poke, sockeye salmon will hold the desired flavor without the meat becoming soft and mushy. Coho salmon (silver) or chinook salmon (king) would be my next choice if sockeye salmon was not available.

Here is what you need to prepare salmon poke:

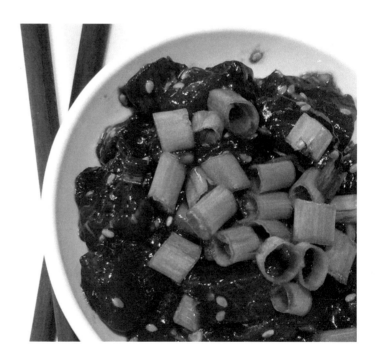

- 1 pound of sashimi grade salmon, cubed in ½ inch pieces

- ½ cup of quality soy sauce (Datu Puti, or low-sodium quality soy sauce)

- 1 bushel of fresh chives

- 1 tablespoon of sesame oil

- 1 teaspoon of fish sauce (use sparely)

- ½ tablespoon of toasted sesame seeds

- ½ tablespoon of crushed red pepper flakes

- 1-2 tablespoons of raw honey

- 2 tablespoons of fresh ginger, minced

Directions: The quality of your salmon and soy sauce is key. After your frozen salmon filet is completely defrosted, you can easily de-bone your filet and cut into ½ inch cubes. Place in medium-size bowl with all other ingredients (following by order of list) and mixed well. Ensure to refrigerate the poke for 2 hours before serving.

CHAPTER 7:

FOR THE SMOKER

If you still cannot get away from eating meat altogether, you can at least make your cooking options a bit healthier by using a smoker. Not everyone is a grill master or smoker savvy, so when purchasing a smoker remember that they come in a variety of sizes and types. In our home, we use an electric smoker, and it is the easiest way to smoke meats without using additional cooking oils. All you need is time, electricity, and wood chips. Some smokers work similarly to a charcoal grill, so you will be able to save on electricity with those. Here are a few smoking techniques to provide healthier options for those people who just cannot get away from eating meat.

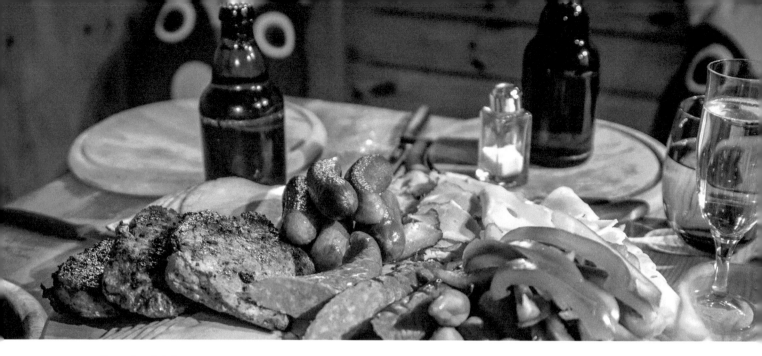

Smoked Meats

Turkey: Next Thanksgiving, give this one a go if you enjoy the process of smoking meats. It is not only a healthier option (than our traditional fried Thanksgiving turkey—yikes!), but I have found this to be a great way to really bring out the turkey flavor. Of course, there are variations of smokers, and wood chips come in a few common flavors like hickory, mesquite, and apple, to name a few. We went with the apple wood chips in an electric upright smoker to smoke up this great holiday favorite.

A twenty-pound or smaller turkey is ideal for the smoking process to really be manageable in terms of maintaining the internal temperature and overall smoking time. You can expect the turkey to be in the smoker for three to four hours.

Preparation is key for turkeys. We like to use a meat injector and a homemade injectable seasoning. For the seasoning, we use melted butter, lemon juice, Tabasco brand hot sauce, powdered garlic, and cayenne pepper. The breast should be generously filled with the liquid seasoning as the white breast meat is usually the driest portion after cooking. After you are satisfied with the amount of flavoring you have pumped into the bird, let it sit covered in your refrigerator for at least twenty-four hours to allow the marinade to work in thoroughly.

While cooking, the **turkey baste** will need to be evenly applied every forty-five minutes. Mix the following together:

- 1 tablespoon of apple cider

- 2–3 tablespoons of raw honey

- 1 cup of chicken stock

Heat the smoker prior to adding the turkey, and set the temperature to 275 degrees. You will need a meat thermometer to ensure that the breast meat reaches 155 degrees and the thigh meat reaches 165 degrees. When those temperatures are reached, the turkey is ready to be removed.

Note: Remember after cooking any type of meat, ensure to let it sit and cool down for at least ten minutes so the juices and seasoning have time to set in.

Venison, Moose, Bison, Pork Ribs: Smoking meats can take as long as your willpower can last. At a minimum, you will need about four to five hours to smoke red meats, but it is critical that the internal temperature reaches 145 degrees. Generally, the longer you can let anything smoke, the more tender the meat will be, but below are a few common time and temperature guidelines for smoking meats in an electric smoker.

Smoking Durations and Temperatures Based on an Electric MasterBuilt Upright Smoker

Meat	Cooking Duration	Temperature
Beef, pork, lamb, veal	4–5 hours	145 degrees F
Pork roast	4–5 hours	145 degrees F
Pork ribs (boneless)	3 1/2 hours	225 degrees F
Pork ribs (baby back)	4 hours	225 degrees F
Deer leg (larger portions) (8 hours total)	6 hours	135 degrees F
	2 hours	140 degrees F

Smoked Salmon: Everyone has his or her own personal technique for smoked salmon, in terms of the actual smoking process. There are a few steps to consider. There is the brine itself; the pellicle, or drying the outer layer of the salmon; then the slow smoking process. For all who use a smoker, I will provide a dry brine and a wet brine recipe here; there is a clear difference in taste and texture based on the two types of brine methods. Also, the type of salmon will determine taste and texture. Of course, everything can be altered to your personal palate, but below is a table of ingredients that are typically used to smoke sockeye salmon.

Wet Brine (for soaking) 24 hours	Dry Brine seasoning for 24 hours
8 cups of water	Light coat of raw honey
2 cups of low-sodium soy sauce	Salt (non-iodized)
1 1/2 cups brown sugar	Powered garlic
1/2 cup salt (non-iodized)	Cayenne pepper
1 1/2 tablespoons garlic powder	Powered ginger
1 tablespoon fresh minced ginger	(Optional) Fish-Seasoning

Once the salmon filets have been in brine of choice for 24 hours, be sure to cut the filets in two-inch wide pieces to ensure smoking duration is sufficient.

Note: For a jerky-like textual for smoked salmon, use the dry brine recipe, cut long ½-inch wide strips and ensure to leave an inch of skin on one end only to "hang" the strips in your smoker. Smoking salmon jerky-strips should take no more than 2 hours on 135 degrees F.

The pellicle phase of smoking salmon is the most important step. This is the phase of drying the salmon meat itself. The duration of

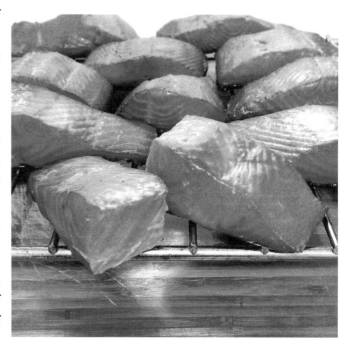

the drying depends on the type of brine you used, the type of salmon species and drying method. Best practices may include pulling the salmon filets out of the low-sodium brine, laying the salmon cut portions out evenly on a wired drying rack tray (skin-side down) and placing an electric fan in front of the trays. When drying is complete, the pellicle texture will feel tacky to the touch. The dryer the salmon meat, the more jerky-like texture you will have after the smoking process.

Smoking duration and temperatures are based on settings for an electric MasterBuilt upright smoker. Again, your type of smoker and the type of salmon will also affect taste and texture.

Type of Salmon	Cooking Duration	Temperature
Silver or king salmon filets (6 hours total)	2 hours	125 degrees F
	2 hours	145 degrees F
	2 hours	165–175 degrees F (depends on filet thickness)
Sockeye salmon filets (5 hours total)	4 1/2 hours	125 degrees F
	30 minutes	135 degrees F
Salmon bellies	4 1/2 hours	135 degrees F
Salmon jerky-strips	1-2 hours	135 degrees F

Octopus

During our annual shrimping and camping trip, we accidentally caught two octopuses in our shrimp pots. An octopus is a cephalopod, which are the largest type of mollusks. These are craziest creatures I have ever caught, as they are extremely fast, intelligent, and absolutely creepy. Octopuses have arms, or tentacles, that are lined with suction cups for gripping and moving around—all very tasty parts to be cooked up in so many different ways.

It is a pretty common occurrence that these amazing sea creatures slither into small spaces by way of changing their bodies' form just to snatch up a bunch of sitting prey, such as the shrimp in our pots! To actually see the two to three-foot tricksters squeeze through a one-inch hole in our shrimp pots was amazing in itself. I have gained so much respect for the octopus and its

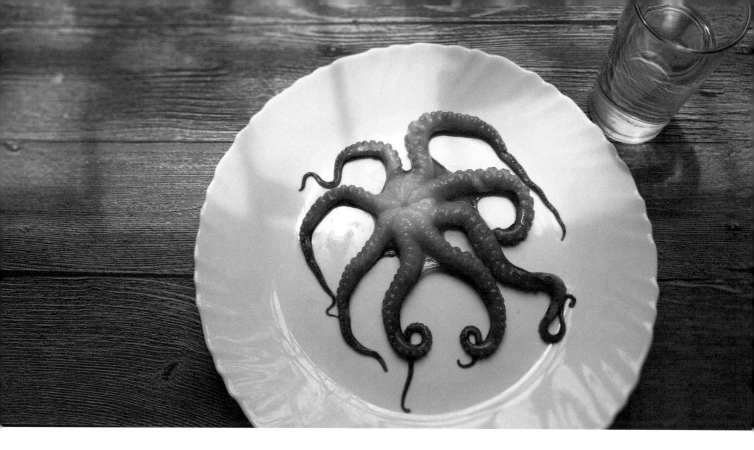

clever tactics. In fact, I could write an entire section on the octopus's ability to move, but what really motivated me to add these cooking methods for octopus was the overwhelming interest on this unique sea creature.

After cleaning the guts out of the massive head, my husband and I harvested about twenty pounds of tentacle meat. I have to give my husband credit for cleaning and preparing the initial boil of the tentacles, as this was the key to making the meat tender. Octopus can easily have a rubbery texture, as you might expect, so boiling it in a seasoned boil for a minimum of forty-five minutes was the first step before further cooking. The seasoning added for the boil was a homemade concoction of salt, cayenne pepper, garlic powder, and black pepper. Honestly, I ask my husband to season our dinner meals all the time as I have grown to love his Cajun palate.

Once you get the texture to your liking and peel the skin off the tentacles, there are so many ways to eat it. We separated the suction cups, or suckers, and used them as salad toppers as they were. The most common recipe I found was a grilled barbecue style, but we decided to cook and prepare it three different ways: smoked, fried, and octopus kimchi.

Smoked

Once the tentacles are skinned, coat them with raw honey and smoke for about four hours. That's it! We use mesquite smoker wood chips, but smoking methods can vary between electric and manual smokers, as well as different flavored wood chips. Although it was great to eat as is and great for adding to your favorite snacking platter.

Fried

We used a seasoned flour and tempura bread crumb for the frying process. Try to use unrefined peanut oil for frying sea foods instead of other cooking oils based on the higher smoke point it provides for deep-frying, as well as the higher monounsaturated fat content, which can reduce your risk for cardiovascular disease. The texture and taste of fried octopus was similar to what you may have experienced with fried calamari. The dipping sauce used was on point! Try a mixture of Sriracha and raw honey for your next fish fry. Dee-lish!

Octopus Kimchi

It is not the authentic Korean-style, fermented cabbage-based kimchi recipe you might expect, but I used similar ingredients and skipped the fermenting process. This was by far my favorite way to eat octopus.

Here is what you need for octopus kimchi:

- 5–6 seasoned and boiled tentacles, chopped into round pieces

- 1 bunch of green onions, minced

- 1/4 cup of fresh ginger, minced

- 2 tablespoons honey

- 1 tablespoon Sriracha sauce

- 1 tablespoon rice vinegar

- 1 tablespoon sesame oil

- 1 splash fish sauce

Directions: In a large sauce pan, boil about 5 cups of water and add the following seasoning to water: salt, cayenne pepper, garlic powder, and black pepper. Boil the tentacles for forty-five minutes, or until tender. Prepare and combine all ingredients listed. The octopus kimchi is ready to eat immediately.

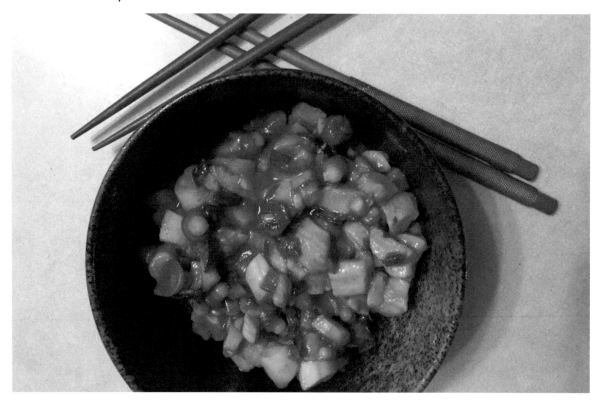

CHAPTER 8:

KEFIR FOR THE WIN!

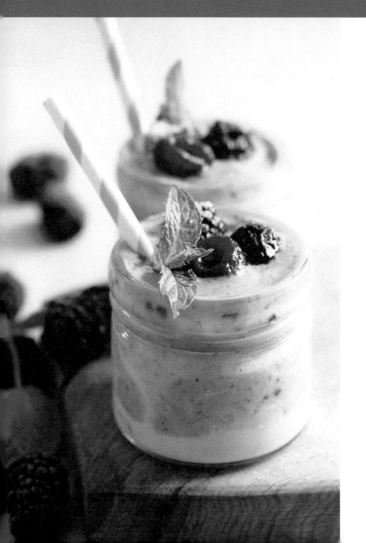

I never thought I would be fermenting milk and feeding it to my children, but I have—for six years now! Seriously, my husband brought kefir grains home after attending a health and fitness course that explained its health benefits. Of course, I couldn't help but do my own research. Now I am hooked on including it in my morning routine and love that my children prefer kefir over store-bought yogurt. Thank goodness too, because store-bought yogurt brands are loaded with sugar, and we all know we get plenty of sugar through other food sources.

Kefir grains are easy to process and can produce a drinkable, yogurt-like beverage or can replace other foods like soft cheese. Any type of milk and time is really all you need. Coconut, almond, and goat's milk can replace your traditional cow's milk, but organic is always the best choice, whether your preference is plant-based or animal milk.

Kefir grains are not grains in the conventional sense but cultures of yeast and lactic acid bacteria that resemble cauliflower in appearance. Over a period of twenty-four hours or so, the microorganisms in the kefir grains multiply and ferment the sugars and preservatives in the milk, turning it into kefir. Then the grains can be removed from the liquid and used over and over again. They multiply quickly and you only need about tablespoon to ferment two cups of milk. So, take what you need and pass the grains on. It is high in nutrients and probiotics and is incredibly beneficial for digestion and gut health. In other words, it's a powerful version of yogurt without the sugars, preservatives, and other additives. It is digestible by those who are lactose intolerant and does not cause breakouts like processed dairy products or conventional store-bought cheese. Finally, there is no added sugar like in many yogurts found in your local grocery store.

Every morning, my kids ask for their fruit smoothies. And the best part of it is that if they leave fruit or vegetable scraps on their plates after any meal, I toss them in a bag in the freezer and throw them in a smoothie the next morning. And the best part, smoothie pops are a cold, sweet snack that kids absolutely love. It is the best way (perhaps the only way) to get my son to eat cucumbers, chia seeds, and spinach. Nothing is wasted in my household, and I try to sneak as many fruits and vegetables in their diets wherever opportunities present. Edamame, spinach, broccoli, cucumbers, apples, oranges, grapes, whatever you can get your kiddos to eat—do not waste these types of fruits and vegetables as they will blend up well in a smoothie.

Here is what you need and the kefir process:

1. Fill a mason jar with kefir grains (which you can buy online) and add 2 cups of your choice of milk. Then cover the jar with cheesecloth and attach the jar ring, allowing the fermenting process to ensue. Let the jar sit in a dark place at room temperature for at least 24 hours. I use a kitchen cabinet to ferment the grains and milk since it will eventually resemble a creepy science experiment on my counter space (eek!).

2. Use a colander to separate the grains from the fermented milk (kefir) and set aside.

3. Fill your blender with the frozen fruit of your choice, spinach or kale, and the fermented kefir. Strawberries, blueberries, and bananas work great; just remember that fruit with seeds will make the smoothie gritty. Pomegranates and raspberries are not recommended

to add to your smoothie based on the seed-like texture. If you add chia seeds, make sure they are softened first by soaking in a liquid of choice overnight.

4. Blend everything together. Hint: adding citrus fruits or raw honey is an easy way to sweeten the smoothie. I commonly add frozen grapes from a previous meal that my children would have left on their plates for waste. No vegetables or fruits should ever go to waste!

5. Use the leftover grains to repeat the fermenting process mentioned above.

Cheers!

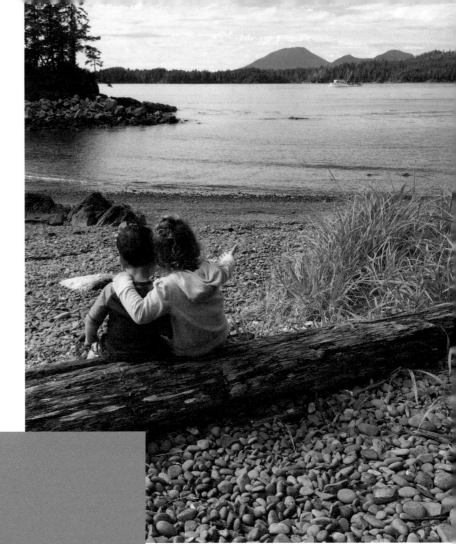

PART 3:

HEALTHY BALANCE THROUGH FOOD AND YOUR ENVIRONMENT

CHAPTER 9:

YOUR LIFESTYLE MATTERS

Despite the obstacles in your life, you still have some control over your moods by eating healthier foods and living an active lifestyle. Understanding your mood triggers and accepting them not as faults or imperfections but rather as a way of how you processed experiences from one time or another is key. What you experienced as a child has the potential to develop mood triggers you may only become aware of as an adult, and you may have a difficult time finding the root of it all. It is also important to understand that you may never fully distinguish one mood trigger from another, but becoming more mindful of them allows you to make better food choices and control your social environment more closely.

I have given you examples through my personal tribulations of moods, food habits, and social environments that have literally shaped me into who I am today. It was not a quick process to figure out the lifestyle that works best for me, and it will not be quick or easy for you either. I can tell you this: being mindful of why you have certain moods and the food you consume can absolutely write or rewrite your future in terms of health status. There are so many things we do today in our lives that will have an impact maybe days, months, or even years later. Simple things, like arguing with a loved one or just listening to a negative person our whole lives has the potential to cause grave damage based on the stress caused by a pointless argument or constant negativity. Such negativity in our lives causes stress on our minds, our hearts, our health, and eventually the people who mean the most to us. Remember, we have the ability to change the food we eat, the people in our lives, and our environment. A strong and supportive community will augment these changes if we find it necessary to overcome stress and depression.

We owe it to ourselves to be mindful of our actions and understand why we have certain mood swings. It is so important to honestly understand ourselves entirely before making sudden and pointless comments or physical actions. Being mindful could change the way people view the world or, more importantly, change the developing path for the children living around us. Everything we do and say is having some impact on our minds and decision processes that essentially define our human behaviors. Becoming more mindful of our thoughts and actions can help us make better decisions and assist us in shaping a healthier lifestyle for ourselves.

Do you like to eat? Perhaps a better question is, do you know what you are eating? A basic rule to follow when you are choosing foods is that if you cannot pronounce all of the ingredients on the label, then you probably should not consume it. The produce aisle is a great place to start for meal planning. Next time you eat a meal, ask yourself if you could visibly recognize and pronounce everything that is listed on the ingredients label or identify all the food on your plate. Certain foods, like products from animals, should be limited in your diet or not consumed at all. At the very least, be mindful of the food processing that took place prior to making it to your table, as I know tasty meats and dairy products can be quite tempting.

And finally, perhaps the most important takeaway we all need to remember is that we are the example for our children. Everything we do and say is being evaluated and tracked as our young children's brains undergo development. As adults, we respond to our environments based on how our brains were hardwired from infancy to adolescence. With that said, parenting has never been so misunderstood as we learn that it is common for adverse child experiences to be a repeating cycle within the family lineage. The environments that children are exposed to are something we as parents can control—for the most part, anyway. Nonetheless, we can definitely provide our children with healthier diets that set them up for success and avoid chronic diseases, such as child obesity, which is currently an American epidemic. We may not be able to change our parents, our experiences, or the exposures we faced as children, but we can certainly make better choices for our children that will support a healthier and more successful outcome in *their* lives. Also, never underestimate the power of love. Showing love and affection to your children is more important than anything else going on in your life. Yes, children are resilient to adverse experiences and can mentally heal from negative experiences, but only if they truly feel loved and are not living in a state of survival. Regardless, it is never too late to take an honest look at your own personal life, understand your mood triggers that may stem from your personal roots, and make better choices for a healthier lifestyle. Specific food choices and daily physical activity will always augment your ability to be more mindful, and mindfulness will help you become a better person.

What Is Your Purpose in Life?

It took courage to publish this book due to its personal content. With my intention to extend a voice to those suffering with depression, PTSD, and chronic health issues, I was not exactly sure this material would hold much value in the public eye. I took the risk and wrote this book anyway because something in my heart told me that some people would relate to my life experiences and possibly make subtle changes in their lives to improve their health. I took the risk of publicly connecting with those who are currently living with fear, confusion, or feelings of worthlessness to relieve some of their stress and remind them that they are not alone in this world. I took a risk to reach out and extend a hand that also holds a wild heart, as we all have different stories to tell and sometimes lose sight of what is really important. We lose sight of the children listening, watching, and learning from us. We forget to pay attention to how we feel after eating and activities we take part in. We forget how many times we ordered takeout this month and how many times we short-changed our diet. We forget to stop and think about what happened in our lives that has the potential to influence our decisions day in and day out. We forget that we are in total control of the environment in which we choose to live and the food we choose to eat.

I provided examples of my personal experiences that shaped my health up to this point in my life. I am still working on identifying personal mood triggers, and I have not found all the answers just yet. More importantly, I am more mindful of my emotions that follow exposures to certain people and events in my life, and I am open to communicate and connect with those people to work through it. I learned, through diet and exercise, that my mood can be altered to a more positive state of mind. I learned to become more mindful of the exposures and experiences I provide for my children for their best and healthiest outcome.

I challenge you to continue to think about your past childhood experiences and any trauma you may have endured in your life. Is there a connection to your unexplained moods? Have you ever really thought about how good or bad you feel after eating certain foods? Have you ever truly listened to the sounds around you during a walk or ever pushed yourself out of your physical and mental comfort zones? Personal growth will open your heart and build your confidence to live a healthier life. Reach out beyond your comfort zone and make those subtle changes. It does not have to be extreme either. There are no super extreme diet and exercise trends to follow or magical pills that help you feel good. Remember, the food and drug industry, health and wellness companies, and the fitness industry are all trying to sell you something. They are all running businesses. Do not fall prey to health-promoting shortcuts when all you really need to do is eat *real* food, drink plenty of water, get plenty of sleep, and enjoy being physically active with something—anything—that gets you moving and more focused. More importantly, become more mindful of yourself and those you love. Stress, depression, and chronic disease are preventable through food and exercise, although life is only truly balanced if you are mentally stable as well.

Our hearts run a course of their own in regard to all things we consider important in life. We all have our own set of priorities and goals, and if your list is short, take the time to mentally revisit your purpose in life. It is too easy to get caught up in what society dictates as important, and so negative thoughts and worthlessness are an easy escape from facing your authentic self. Do not allow society or socioeconomic status define what you are capable of becoming, and never accept that you are not enough in this world. Wild heart, healthy life.

WORKS CITED

American Academy of Pediatrics. 2014. "Adverse Childhood Experiences and the Lifelong Consequences of Trauma." *American Academy of Pediatrics: Dedicated to the Health of all Children.* February 2. https://www.aap.org/en-us/Documents/ttb_aces_consequences.pdf.

ASPCA. 2019. *Factory Farms: Farm Animals Need Our Help.* January 1. Accessed February 5, 2019. https://www.aspca.org/animal-cruelty/farm-animal-welfare.

CDC. 2016. *CDC 24/7: Saving Lives, Protecting People.* December 15. Accessed February 1, 2019. https://www.cdc.gov/obesity/childhood/causes.html.

—. 2018. *Centers of Disease Control and Prevention: Overweight and Obesity, Data and Statistics.* August 13. Accessed February 1, 2019. https://www.cdc.gov/obesity/data/childhood.html.

—. 2018. *Mental Health Conditions: Depression and Anxiety.* March 22. Accessed April 10, 2018. https://www.cdc.gov/tobacco/campaign/tips/diseases/depression-anxiety.html.

—. 2017. *National Center for Statistics: Leading Causes of Death.* Centers for Disease Control and Prevention. March 17. Accessed February 5, 2019. https://www.cdc.gov/nchs/fastats/leading-causes-of-death.htm.

Fairgrieve, William T., and Micheal B. Rust. 2003. "Interactions of Atlantic Salmon in the Pacific Northwest V. Human Health and Safety." *Fisheries Research* 62 (2003): 329-338.

Find a Workout Plan. 2019. *Bodybuilding.com.* January 1. Accessed February 1, 2019. https://www.bodybuilding.com/workout-plans/.

Fox, Maggie. 2010. *Reuters.* Edited by Health Science Editor Maggie Fox. Science News. August 3. Accessed January 1, 2019. https://www.reuters.com/article/us-usa-supplements-idUSTRE6721F520100803.

Freeland, Amber. 2019. *The Cooper Institute: Well. Into the Future.* Kenneth H. Cooper. January 28. Accessed January 29, 2019. http://www.cooperinstitute.org/2019/01/28/healthy-children-today-better-workforce-tomorrow.

Gahche, Jaime, Vicki Burtl, Jeffery Hughes, Regan Bailey, Elizabeth Yetley, Johanna Dwyer, Mary Frances Picciano, Christopher Sempos, and Margaret McDowell. 2011. "Dietary supplement use among U.S. adults has increased since NHANES III (1988–1994)." *Dietary Supplement Use Among U.S. Adults Has Increased Since NHANES III (1988–1994).* April 13. Accessed February 5, 2019. https://www.cdc.gov/nchs/data/databriefs/db61.htm.

Good, Thomas P., Jeremy Davies, Brian J. Burke, and Mary H. Ruckelshaus. 2008. "Incorporating Catastrophic Risk Assessments into Setting Conservation Goals for Threatened Pacific Salmon." *Ecological Applications* 18 (1): 246-257.

Gunders, Dana. 2017. *Wasted: How America Is Losing Up to 40 Percent of Its Food from Farm to Fork to Landfill.* August 16. Accessed January 2019. https://www.nrdc.org/sites/default/files/wasted-food-IP.pdf.

Harvard T.H. Chan. 2019. *Harvard T.H. Chan, School of Public Health: The Nutrition Source.* School of Public Health Harvard T.H. Chan. January 1. Accessed February 5, 2019. https://www.hsph.harvard.edu/nutritionsource/2015/11/03/report-says-eating-processed-meat-is-carcinogenic-understanding-the-findings/.

Johnson, Mike Kissel, and Brad Hubbard. 2019. *Mission 22: United in the War Against Veteran Suicide.* Elderheart Inc. Accessed February 2019. https://www.mission22.com/about/.

Lall, Santosh P. 2010. "The Health Benefits of Farmed Salmon: Fish Oil Decontamination Processing Removes Persistent Organic Pollutants." *British Journal Nutrition* 103 (March): 1391-1392.

Lara, Jose J., Maria Economou, A. Michael Wallace, Anne Rumley, Gordon Lowe, Christine Slater, Muriel Caslake, Naveed Sattar, and Michael E.J. Lean. 2006. "Benefits of Salmon eating on Traditional and Novel Vascular Risk Factors in Young, Non-Obese Healthy Subjects." 193: 213-221.

Mercola, Joseph M. 2010. *Mercola: Take Control of Ypur Health.* Dr. Mercola's Natural Health Newsletter. April 20. Accessed January 1, 2019. https://articles.mercola.com/sites/articles/archive/2010/04/20/sugar-dangers.aspx.

Moore, Jonathan W., Daniel E. Schindler, Jackie L. Carter, Justin Fox, Jennifer Griffiths, and Gordon W. Holtgrieve. 2007. "Biotic Control of Stream Fluxes: Spawning Salmon Drive Nutrient and Matter Export." *Ecology* 88 (5): 1278-1291.

Naiman, Robert J., Robert E. Bilby, Daniel E. Schindle, and James M. Helfield. 2002. "Pacific Salmon, Nutrients, and the Dynamics of Freshwater and Riparian Ecosystems." *Ecosystems* 5 (4): 399-417.

Szalay, Jessie. 2015. *Live Science.* May 13. Accessed February 6, 2019. https://www.livescience.com/50818-kale-nutrition.html.

Tom, Pamela D., and Paul G. Olin. 2010. *Better to Eat - Farmed or Wild Salmon?* May 1. https://www.aquaculturealliance.org/advocate/better-to-eat-farmed-or-wild-salmon/.

PHOTOGRAPHY CITED

1. Table of various food choices https://pixabay.com/en/salad-fruits-berries-healthy-2756467/

2. https://pixabay.com/en/paprika-salad-orange-3212148/ Food pic for bottom of section

3. Mood trigger beginning section photo https://pixabay.com/en/cutout-shape-heart-shutter-wood-212016/

4. Spices in Jar: https://pixabay.com/en/spices-jar-cooking-rustic-pepper-2548653/

5. Raised Garden 1, Raised Garden 2: photos by author

6. Sugars https://pixabay.com/en/sugar-sweets-black-background-2263618/

7. Fruit https://pixabay.com/en/fruit-fruits-fruit-salad-fresh-bio-2305192/

8. Fruit https://pixabay.com/en/berries-raspberries-fruit-fruits-1546125/

9. Journal https://pixabay.com/en/black-coffee-coffee-cup-desk-drink-2847957/

10. Fat oils https://pixabay.com/en/olive-oil-salad-dressing-cooking-968657/

11. Salmon run https://pixabay.com/en/salmon-fish-run-jump-upstream-1107404/

12. Soup and vegetables https://pixabay.com/en/soup-vegetables-pot-cooking-food-1006694/

13. Harvest https://pixabay.com/en/vegetables-vegetable-basket-harvest-752153/

14. Canned sea asparagus, Self-harvest Challenge 1, Self-harvest Challenge 2, Self-harvest Challenge 3: photos by author

15. Salmon berry: photo by author

16. Squash https://pixabay.com/en/butternut-squash-butternut-squash-3597762/

17. Cucumber salad: photo by author

18. Cumber Kimchi: photo by author

19. Halibut ceviche https://pixabay.com/en/ceviche-menu-shrimp-639900/

20. Kale https://pixabay.com/en/kale-swiss-chard-arugula-vegetable-1775809/

21. Kale salad with apples: photo by author

22. Lemon and Honey https://pixabay.com/en/fresh-fruit-health-healthcare-3533085/

23. Costa Rica Salad: photo by author

24. Squash soup: photo by author

25. Vegetable Pho https://pixabay.com/en/pho-vietnamese-food-restaurant-263127/

26. Shrimp Pho https://pixabay.com/en/tom-yum-goong-hot-and-sour-soup-1216817/

27. Salmon Poke: photo by author

28. Smoked Food Platter https://pixabay.com/photos/jause-eat-delicious-food-338498/

29. Smoked Salmon: photo by author

30. Octopus Plate https://pixabay.com/en/food-plate-delicious-meal-3556782/

31. Octopus Kimchi: photo by author

32. Kefir https://pixabay.com/en/cocktail-breakfast-fruit-2295728/

33. Boy and Girl Beach: photo by author.